BLOOD PURIFIER
IN
UNANI MEDICINE

Dr. Ansari Mushir

MD (NIUM BANGALORE)
BUMS (MIJT MUMBAI)
PGDEMS (LIHS MUMBAI)

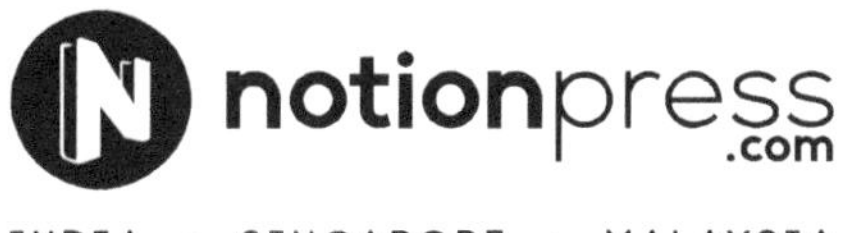

INDIA • SINGAPORE • MALAYSIA

ISBN 000-0-00000-000-0

Contents

Preface

The concept of blood purifier drugs is unique. These drugs are endowed with a number of pharmacological actions. An extensive search was carried out for this book to record all the available information in Unani literature on the concepts of blood, impure blood and blood purification. Unani classical books of different languages and discussion with experts were conferred with for this book. Contemporary reference books, relevant articles, peer reviewed indexed journals were assessed to find out on going current theories and advancement in the field of herbal medicine. This book may serve as a tool for a student, teachers, medical practitioner as well as common man seeking guidance in the field of blood purification by herbal drugs. Various scientific studies on blood purifier drugs on various common human diseases and different blood purifier medicine available in the market are also included in this book which helps Unani, Ayurvedic and Allopathic practitioner to treat diseases.

ACKNOWLEDGMENT

I started to write this book in the year 2019 but because of diligent duties it got delayed.

I thank Almighty Allah for provididing me the knowledge, strength and ability to write this book.

I dedicate this book to my parents Mrs. Shakira and Mr. Akhtar, my family Dr Sabah my daughter Zainab and son Saad.

I would like to express my heartly gratitude to my Teacher, my guide, my mentor Prof Dr. Nasreen Jahan without her help this would not be possible.

My sincere thanks and love to my family, friends, teachers, staff and students for the unconditional encourangment throughout this work.

Blood Purifiers In Unani System of Medicine

UNANI MEDICINE: RIVER OF KNOWLEDGE

Unani medicine a distinctive medical system began since two thousand years ago. The system is well structured and established on plausible and scientific theories. The concept of Unani system of medicine is unique. The concepts of blood purifier, aphrodisiacs, organ-specific tonics, immunomodulators, etc. are exclusive features of this system.

Many of its theories and principles are different from that of Western medicine and these theories have been proposed by an outstanding scholar of the ancient era, like Hippocrates, Galen, Avicenna etc. The basic physiology of Unani medicine revolves around seven fundamental factors viz. *arkān* (Elements), *mizāj* (Temperament), *akhlāt* (Humours), *a'da'* (Organs), *arwāh* (Vital force), *quwā* (Faculties) and *af'al* (Functions). Humoral theory is the backbone of this system, remarkable for explaining various functions of the body ranging from providing nutrition to beautification of the body. According to Hippocrates, when the four *akhlāt* (Humours) *viz. dam* (sanguine), *balgham* (phlegm), *safrā'* (yellow bile) and *sawdā'* (black bile) are properly mingled, the body is in a state of health, but when there is dyscrasia or disequilibrium in the mixtures, disease arises.

Blood in Unani Literature

Since ancient times, blood has been accredited as the vital component of life. Without knowledge of the circulation, ancient Egyptians recognized the heart as the seat of the soul. The ancient philosophers agreed about blood and its function and their views were upheld for almost two thousand years. Galen (131-201 AD) and Celsus (25 BC-50 AD) summarized these beliefs in their respective books. In the fifteenth century, blood was optional for fits, melancholia, lunacy, palsy and bad disposition. Blood is regarded as a mixture of all four *Akhlāt* viz. *Dam, balgham, safrā'* and *sawdā'*. Since *dam* is superior in all *khilṭ* and red colour is dominated in the blood hence, the whole mixture is called as *dam* or *khūn*. *Atibba* use these two terms synonymously. *Dam* is considered best among all *khilt*. It provides nutrition to the body as well as *badl ma yatahallal* (replacement of wear and tear) whenever the nourishment is lost. This replacement is equal to the sum of wear and tear in adults and the replacement is more in growing age and less in old age. Further Abu Sahal Masihi (960-1000 AD) has defined that "*Tabi'i khūn* is one in which all *akhlāt* are in normal proportion both in *kayfiyat* and *kammiyat*". It should be normal in colour, free from bad odour, moderate in viscosity and taste, free from *ufūnat* and *humūdat*. Blood is considered as heterogeneous fluid as nearly all *akhlāt* participates into its composition. Moreover the ancient physicians have also described *akhlāt latifah* (fine humors) and *akhlāt kathifa* (coarse humor), which could be attributed to liquid part and cellular elements, respectively.

The *qiwam* (viscosity) of the normal blood is *mu'tadil* (normal) in thinness and thickness and it is an important property of blood. The viscosity of blood depends on the quantity of humours and tension of *al bukharate dukhaniya* (carbon dioxide) in the blood. It is why Al Abbas (died 994 AD), claims that the *qiwam* (viscosity) of arterial blood is lower than the venous blood.

Production of Blood

According to Avicenna, all the four humours are primarily derived from the metabolism of food and utilized as nutrient components for growth, maintenance and repair of the organs and to yield energy for the work. Accoridng Razi Blood is distributed to all the organs through the vessels to fulfill their different requirements. As soon as food enters the mouth, teeth start crushing it and tongue helps in mixing the food items with saliva. Parts of food get digested in mouth before reaching the stomach where remaining process of digestion takes place. Simultaneously *qalb* (heart) also plays an important role though indirectly in digestion through its *harārat gharīziyya* (innate heat/natural heat). It helps not only in distribution of food particles to the body parts but also helps in their assimilation (*tagairaah*). After gastric and intestinal digestion, food turns into chyme and chyle. *Ma'sareqa* (mesenteric vessels) and the branches of the portal vein (*warid al-bab*) absorb the food from gut and carry it to the liver where hepatic digestion takes place; chyle is converted into four humours in varying quantities, blood being the largest. Unani physicians hold the opinion that most of the metabolic functions take place in liver whereas the modern medicine argues that various useful substances are formed in liver which directly or indirectly controls the heamatopoeisis. According to the Northern blot analysis, the liver and kidneys appear to be the major sites of thrombopoietin mRNA expression. The findings of a study demonstrate that liver is the major site of thrombopoietin (Tpo) production and altered hepatic Tpo production will lead to a significant reduction in platelet levels. Further, biological assay of the human liver in various types of anaemia also showed conspicuous differences in the concentration of haemoglobin producing factors. The sinuses of liver can release several hundred milliliters of blood into circulation. Now it is clear that most part of the blood and its components like black bile, yellow bile and phlegm are produced in liver that is why Nafis (15th cent AD) stated that, "Normal blood is one which is formed and processed to purity in the liver". However, presently it may explain the haemopoiesis during mid trimester of gestation. Guyton describes hepatic macrophage system as the blood-cleansing system which is also carried at hepatic level. Blood flowing in intestinal capillaries picks up many bacteria from the intestines. A sample of blood taken from the portal veins, before it enters the liver, almost always grows colon bacilli when cultured, Kupffer cells, the large phagocytic macrophages cleanse blood in less than 0.01 second; the bacterium passes inward through the wall of the Kupffer cell to become permanently lodged inside until it is digested. Blood is mostly produced with hot and moist food such as *lahm* (meat). This has been accepted by the contemporary physiology, that meat contains first class proteins i.e. essential amino acids which are essential for formation of haemoglobin and help in the production of plasma protein (Whipple 1940). The stomach protein and nucleoprotein of the blood corpuscles are also formed with these first class proteins.

CHARACTERISTICS OF BLOOD

Blood is considered a heterogeneous fluid because almost all humours participate in its composition. However, the broad division of composition includes *akhlāt latifah* (fine parts of humours) and *akhlāt kathifa* (coarse parts of humours) and may be taken as correlates of liquid part and cellular elements respectively as described by modern physiology. *Akhlāt kathifa* have barid kaifiyat predominant and take part in assimilation by the organ while *akhlāt latifah* have *har kaifiyat* predominant and carry out vital function and are dynamic. Here an analogy to the heavier part of blood is referred to *Kaseef akhlat* like RBC, WBC etc. and lighter part to *lateef akhlat* like plasma. The best parts of all humours are supposed to be intermingled in blood. Yellow bile maintains the viscosity of blood and makes it *latif* (diffusible), the black bile provides mass and thickness to the blood due to which the blood is retained in its place and the phlegm makes the blood sticky. All these humours are attributable to the primordial importance of blood as these components are intermingled with it and the body organs take their required nutrition from the blood.

The desired *qiwam* (viscosity) of blood considered as one of its important properties is *mu'tadil* (normal) indicating that it is equiponderantin thinness and thickness. The viscosity of blood depends on the quantity of humours and tension of *al bukharate dukhaniya* (carbon dioxide) in the blood. That is why Al Abbas (994 AD) claimed that the *qiwam* (viscosity) of arterial blood is lower than the venous blood. The ancient physicians had explained the coexistence of four humours in the body with the help of its physical property of sedimentation. They reported that when the *fasd* (venesection) was performed and blood was taken in a bowl, its heavier part settled down soon. Due to this sedimentation, four layers of blood were seen. The uppermost layer which was the thinnest of all, devoid of any corpuscle and bore yellow colour was called yellow bile. Below the layer of yellow bile was a denser and white layer lacking any corpuscles was called as phlegm; below this layer was a relatively heavier layer of red colour consisting of corpuscles was called as *dam*. The lowermost layer was heaviest of all and contained all heavier compounds and packed deoxygenated red blood corpuscles exhibiting dark blackish colour. Due to its dark or blackish colour it was called black bile. When blood is shed, it quickly loses its fluidity and sets into semisolid jelly. This phenomenon is called as coagulation. The coagulated blood if kept further for sometime retracts to a smaller volume and passes out a straw coloured fluid called as *masal-al-dam* (serum). The phenomenon of *injimādal dam* (coagulation of blood) was well known to the ancient physicians. Abu Sahal Masihi (960-1000 AD) called the threads of fibrin of clot as *"khoyoot"* and suggested *hābis-i-dam* (coagulants and styptics) agents to arrest bleeding. It has been mentioned that intravascular clotting is prevented by the role of *tabiat* (physics) or the structure of vessels. This has also been accepted by modern scientists who suggested that in vessels, there are some protective substances which protect blood from clotting. A healthy vessel produces vasoactive hormones known as nitric oxide and prostacyclin. Both nitric oxide and prostacyclin relax blood vessels and inhibit platelet activation thus prevent intravascular coagulation. Coagulation depends on various factors (chemical compounds) present in the blood. Deficiency in any of these factors causes *su'almizāj* (dyscrasia) in the blood leading to haemorrhage or delay in coagulation which may derange the haemostatic mechanism of the body.

Ancient physicians have tried to describe the quantity of *dam* in the body and its actual share in total humoural fluid. A group of Unani scholars is of the view that *dam* is half of total humoural quantity followed by black bile, phlegm and yellow bile. According to Nafis (15th cent. AD) the authentic statement in this regard is that of Abu Sahal Masihi (960-1000 AD), who said that black bile is found minimally in the composition. Hence most of the physicians reckoned that the quantity of *dam* is high followed by phlegm, yellow bile and black bile. *Mizaj* (temperament) is a unique concept of Unani medicine as the functions of organs/tissues depend on or mediated through it. The temperament of blood has been described to be *hār ratab* (hot and moist) which assumes significance because of its widespread occupancy in the body. *Harārat* (heat) of blood indicates that some of its constituents participate in the production of heat which in turn helps in maintaining the body temperature and keeps certain variables of the body in equilibrium. This is mainly achieved through blood plasma which absorbs or give off heat and through the speed at which the blood flows. When the blood vessels expand, the blood flows slowly which causes heat to be lost and vice versa. Unani scholars have given reasons for the verification of the temperament of blood for example, if it is formed by the foods of hot and moist temperament like meat, alcohol and dates etc.; then the blood causes hot wet diseases like *humma mutbiqa* (continuous fever) which is cured by drugs of opposite temperament i.e. *bārid yābis* (cold and dry) medicine. The hot temperament of blood reflects on the realization that the organs which are highly supplied by blood are hot while those having poor blood supply are either less hot or cold. Further, if the supply of blood of an organ is seized the organ becomes extremely cold and even death of the part occurs soon.

Another reason of its hotness is that it maintains the body at a uniform temperature and keeps the viscera warm to perform their normal function. Blood contains many constituents which are potentially hot e.g. when they reach the organs; they are oxidized to produce heat and energy. It is *ratab* (wet) because of the presence of moist substances in it which accounts for 91-92% of the total blood, that is why it produces such signs and symptoms in the body which are attributed to *rutūbat* (wet/moist substances).

Functions of Blood

The functions of blood explained by ancient physicians are more or less same as described in modern physiology. According to various eminent Unani scholars, blood gives nutrition and helps in growth of organs and body. Almost similar description has been given by Western medicine where it has been mentioned that nutrients derived from the digested food materials i.e.glucose, amino acids, lipids, etc. are absorbed from the alimentary canal and carried by blood to tissues for their growth. It provides *harārat gharīzi* (innate heat) to various organs through the arteries arising from the heart. It also provides energy and helps in replacement of wear and tear. According to conventional medicine, blood flow is required for healing and maintenance and growth of body cells. Further, it has been elucidated that changes in blood flow rate affect growth of cell population and if blood supply further decreases, cells may die. One of the life saving functions of blood described in Unani text is that it keeps the body warm. This is also similar to functions stated in modern physiology indicating that blood regulates body temperature through high specific heat, high thermal conductivity, high latent heat of vaporization and quick flow. According to Unani physician, blood makes the skin lustrous, red, attractive and beautiful. Blood flow nourishes the skin cells and keeps them lively. Blood flow also carries away waste products and toxic substances including free radicals from working cells thus keeps skin healthy and lovely. Blood provides *madda* (material) for the genesis of *a'da' mutashabiha* (homogeneous organs) and acts as *hamile ruh* (carrier of oxygen). It serves as a link between individual cells of distant organs and tissues.

Types of Blood

Ismail Jurjani (1041-1136 AD) has classified blood into two categories. First one is red and somewhat viscous, found in liver and vessels arising from it. Other is bright red present in heart and in the vessels arising from the heart. Other physicians have divided blood into two different types i.e. normal and abnormal. Unani scholars have mentioned a few physical qualities of normal blood in respect of its colour, taste, smell, viscosity etc. Colour of blood is red though the shades of arterial and venous blood vary a little. Ali Ibn Abbas Majoosi (died 982–994 AD) stated that the colour of arterial blood is scarlet red and vein is dark red. Blood is sweet in taste as sweet substances similar to grape juice are found in the composition of blood in large quantity. But when changes occur in its quality it becomes sweet as alcohol. Because of its sweetness, organs absorb blood easily in required quantity. Some of the salty substances have also been described to be present in the blood which are considered beneficial for the body. It dissolves excessive phlegm and prevents blood from *ufūnat* (sepsis). Normal blood is odourless but some of the scholars have mentioned about the presence of odour in the blood. However, it has been stated that blood should be free from bad odour because it is a clear sign of sepsis. Bad smell of blood is associated with *humudat* (acidity) which is mainly caused due to fermentation, a correlate of sepsis. Blood should be normal in viscosity. Blood with normal viscosity provides nutrition to both hollow and dense organs and the *ruh* (pneuma) can be formed from it. If a person's blood is normal in quantity and quality, then he looks happy and all his activities are in order. But when it is altered somehow the alteration in temperament of blood takes place leading to a reduction in the oxygen carrying capacity of the blood. As a result, organs are affected badly which further disturb the temperament of blood. This causes deranged body functions i.e. diseases.

Causes of Production of Ghayr tabi'i Dam

If we go right back to early history, it will be appreciated that various terms such as "thick blood", "thin blood", "too much blood", "too litle blood", "dirty blood", "bad blood" etc. have been commonly used in the ancient manuscripts. Abu Sahal Masihi (960-1000 AD) an eminent scholar of Unani medicine, has mentioned that normal blood is one in which all humours are in normal proportion both in terms of quality and quantity. Proper functioning of stomach, liver, kidney and spleen is necessary for the production of good quality of blood. A well known philosopher Ibn Rushd (1126 –1198 AD.) has described that temperament of organs remains normal when the blood which nourishes them is normal in quantity and quality. Unhealthy food, irregular dietary habit, unhealthy environment, stressing occupation etc. may contribute to produce morbid blood. Foods responsible for blood dyscrasia include salty, spicy and rotten stuffs etc. People with grueling and stressful job are more prone to acquire blood dyscrasia. Sometimes, a combination of both internal and external causes, leads to the production of humour which is abnormal in terms of both, the quality and quantity.

According to Unani concepts the functional disturbance of liver following a change in its mizäj (temperament), affects the production of blood as such and alters its normal composition and the quality. The proper functioning of spleen which is necessary to maintain the physiology of blood is also modified. If spleen fails to clean the blood having undesirable barid yäbis (cold dry) substances then mizaj of liver becomes abnormal drifting to barudat (coldness) and yäbusat (dryness). In case of sue mizäj yäbis of the liver the viscosity of blood increases while its volume decreases, whereas in sue mizäj ratb (abnormal wet temperament) of liver the volume of blood increases. However, excessive abnormal harärat (vital heat) i.e. sue mizäj här (abnormal hot temperament) can cause debility in liver function, as a result liver may be unable to produce normal constituents of blood. According to Ibn Sina (980-1037AD), blood becomes morbid under the influence of sue mizäj säda (qualitative altered temperament). It has been further argued that blood becomes morbid because of the intervention of two main factors: either because of pathological components of external environment or morbid substances produced endogenously. When a component part of blood becomes muta‘affin (septic) its lateef (diffusible) part is changed into serous bile and kaseeef (coarse) part into bilious melanchole, whereas the second variety in which temperament is changed by morbid humour, has several sub types depending on involvement of specific humour and the types of morbid humour e.g. various types of phlegm, black bile, or yellow bile.

Pathological Aspect

Changes occurring in blood that convert it in to abnormal blood vary enormously depending upon the pathological component involved. Blood may become viscous, morbid, and serous, or its taste may change into bitter, salty or sour. Morbid blood also varies in colour. The colour may be blackish or bluish or whitish. Whitish colour which is the reflection of coldness appears to be due to dominance of phlegm which has colder temperament as compared to the normal blood. Black colour is the expression of ascendance of black bile or a demonstration of ihteraq combustion/oxidation) of other humours; it is warmer than blood predominant with other excessive humours. Smell of blood may become abnormal due to access of any mut'affin khilt (infected humour) or due to ta'affun (sepsis) in blood itself. The taste of morbid blood changes in commensuration of the specific. Excess humor is the major cause of morbidity. It becomes bitter due to yellow bile or sour due to balgham hamiz (sour phlegm) or sawdä' hamiz (sour melanchole). Blood becomes abnormally viscous due to inordinate amount of phlegm and serous due to presence of excessive yellow bile (Table 1& 2). On the basis of these changes morbid blood are classified into fourteen different types Ismail Jurjani (1041-1136 AD) has given a detailed account of morbid blood in his book Zakheera Khwarzam Shahi. According to him khün safrä'wi (bilious sanguine) is less viscous than normal, yellowish in colour, strong in odour, frothy, hotter, takes much time to coagulate and is relatively bitter in taste. Khün balghami (phlegmatic sanguine) when exposed outside the body it is soggy but very soon it becomes viscous, coagulates in a very short time and has mild odour, but if infected it causes to emit bad odour and when kept for an hour it releases fluid. Whereas khün sawdä'wi (melancholic sanguine) is black, viscous and has bad odour. It does not take much time to coagulate. If a little water is added to it and shaken, it scatters and takes the shape of fibers and liberates bluish watery fluid (Table 1 & 2).

Abnormal Blood in Contemporary Perspective

No emphasis has been laid on colour, taste and smell of blood to describe its quality character as such or as correlates of pathological manifestation in conventional medicine, whereas Unani physicians have described specific colour, taste and smell of normal blood. Unani medicine also stated that a change in colour of blood leads to change in the colour of skin and urine. Examination of urine and skin is still considered an important tool in the diagnosis of different diseases. There is no mention of hematological diseases categories in ancient Unani classics that exactly correspond to modern classification; however, it does not imply that Unani medicine has not been confronted with hematological diseases. Pathological changes that occur in hematological diseases may be correlated with morbid blood, as the signs and symptoms of blood diseases as described in modern medicine are almost similar to that of morbid blood. Splenomegaly is the crucial diagnostic sign in most of the diseases of blood. Interestingly Unani physicians have mentioned that in case of spleenenlargement, body in general and liver in particular become weak, as a result liver shows insufficiency to produce normal blood. Moreover, spleen absorbs extra amount of blood which leads to further shortage of blood. Symptoms of fatigue, weakness, tiredness and fever were described by ancient physicians under amrad' tihäl (splenic diseases) and almost similar symptoms are mentioned in conventional medicine under caption of various hematological disorders.

Though abnormality in any of the humour is responsible for morbid blood but excess of black bile is considered as the leading cause. The excess of black bile produces anaemia because it stagnates in between the liver and stomach and thereby interferes with the production of blood and humors. The diseases such as abnormal cold temperament of liver, stomach or intestine or hemorrhage etc cause commotion in the function of liver, especially its hematopoietic activity is altered. One of the study concluded that in patients with massive splenomegaly with ascites and cirrhosis, investigation should be focused on haematological diseases. This indicates that hematological diseases may manifest in the form of splenomegaly and ascites. Unani physicians in their treatises declared that su ul qinya (a complex disease involving mainly liver and spleen and causing severe anaemia) leads to ascites (Fig.1).

Characteristics	**Unani medicine**
Colour	scarlet red (arterial) dark red (venous)
Odour	Odourless/devoid of bad odour
Temperament	Hot
Viscosity	Moderately viscous
Taste	Sweet
Reaction	Alkaline
Quantity	Highest in proportion to other *khilt*

Diseases and Blood

Garm tar māddī diseases occur due to mild alteration in quantity and quality of blood as severe alteration may transform blood into other *khilṭ*. At this situation the converted *khilṭ* is only accountable for the disease. The diseases caused by abnormal blood are predominantly *ḥumma* and *waram*. *Hummiyat damwi* or *ḥumma mutbiqa* (continuous fever) may be *ghalayānī* or *ufūni*. Ghalayān (synochus fever) caused by *ghalayān* of blood in the region of liver and heart without sepsis or accumulation of hot vapour. Reason for josh and *ghalayān khūn* is sudda formed by excessive *khūn* which decreases the *harārat* ghariziyya thereby *harārat* ghariba increased which agitates *khūn* and leads to josh in it. Sometimes the cause of josh is severe *ḥumma* yaum. Sometimes sepsis may occur due to *harārat* which converts into *ḥumma mutbiqa* or because of decreased viscosity may transform into *sarsām* (meningitis) or *judarī* (small pox). Humma *ufūni* (septic fever) arises due to sepsis at inside or outside vessels. If it is inside then known as haqiqi while in case of other, fever is caused by damwi waram.

Falghamuni is a type of *waram* caused by increased quantity of blood. When supplying blood of any organ becomes *ghayr mu'tadil* in its quality the *warm* produced known as *jamra khalsa* (carbuncle), *judarī* (small pox), *hasba* (small pox), *awram hadda* (acute inflammation), some types of gout is also included in *awram damwiyya* caused by impurity or infection in blood. *Humma damwiyya* is necessary with these diseases. It may be fatal if the blood becomes severely *fasid*. *Akhlāt raddiyya* are always painful whether they altered quantitatively or qualitatively e.g. *Akhlāt ladha'*(burning) due to *sue mizāj* or excessive *khilṭ* causes congestion and leads to *tafarruq-i-ittisal*. Arastu stated that when blood becomes impure it migrates towards nose or anus and bleeding starts from there therefore impure blood may be considered as one of the causes of bleeding disorders.

The author of *Kitabul Umda fil Jarahat* was well aware of diseases caused by *fasade dam*. He compiled one chapter by the name "disease caused by *fasade khūn* include *falghamuni* (sanguineous inflammation), *judari, dummal* (boil), *banāt al-layl* (urticaria), *dakhis* (paronychia), *ta'un* and *anurasma* (aneurysm). Its surgical treatment has been described in detail.

Some disorders of blood are specific to vessels e.g. bleeding due to opening of the pores of vessels. It may be due to the malfunction of *quwwat dafi'a* or diseases of vessels itself e.g. *tafarruq-i-ittisal* of vessels occurs due to *hiddat, riqqat* and *latafat* of *khūn.* Sometime with excessive quantity of blood the quality of blood is also altered it is called *imtila bahasbal quwa.* But if changes occur only in *kayfiyat* cause disturbances in *quwate jismani* leads to anorexia, weakness/ lethargy simply it can be said that all *af'al nafsaniya* and *tabiya* become weak and lethargic. But signs and symptoms of *imtila bahsabal tajaweef* is different.

Table 1: Characteristics of Tabi‘i and Ghayr Tabi‘i Dam

Characteristics	**Tabi‘i dam**	**Ghayr tabi‘i dam**
Colour	Red	Blackish /Bluish / Whitish
Odour	Odourless/devoid of bad odour	Bad odour
Temperament	*Hārr ratab*	Altered
Viscosity	*Motadil*	Viscous/Watery
Taste	Sweet	Bitter /Sour/Salty
Reaction	Alkaline	Acidic
Quantity	Highest in proportion to other *khilṭ*	Altered

Table 2: Characteristics of Ghayr Tabi'i Dam due to Dominance of Khil

Characteristics	***Safrā***	***Sawdā'***	***Balgham***
Colour	Yellowish	Blackish	Whitish
Appearance	Frothy	-	-
Odour	Strong	Bad/Sour	Mild
Viscosity	Less viscous	More viscous	Viscous and Sticky
Taste	Bitter	Sour	Sour
Coagulation time	Delayed	Moderate	Early
Temperament	Excessive hot	Excessive hot	Less hot

Importance of Tanqiya Khūn

All parts of food can't become nutrition but some waste and bad things remains inside body. If these waste materials become excessive they can lead to various types of diseases. There are various organs and ways in the body by which these morbid humours are removed.[9] The importance of *tanqiya khūn* can be appreciated when gall bladder fails to absorb *mirra safrā'* and *mirra safrā'* coalesce with blood then different type of *safrā'wi* diseases can occur like *yarqan* (jaundice), *buthur labaniyya* (acne), *jamra* (carbuncle), *namla* (herpes) etc. Likewise when spleen is unable to absorb *sawdā'wi khilṭ* and that *khilṭ* coalesce with blood, disease like *yaraqan aswad* (jaundice), *bahaq aswad* (pitryasis nigra), *quba* (ring worm/dermatophytosis), *niqris* (gout), *namash* (naevus), *judham* (leprosy), *malankhuliya* (melancholia) etc. evolved. Similarly if kidneys are unable to absorb excessive water from liver blood diseases like *Istisqa lahmi* (cachexic oedema/anasarca.), *istisqa ziqqi* (ascites.) can develop. It can be concluded that if these three *fuzalat* are not absorbed properly by their absorbing organs then human body will always be in diseased state.[9]

Treatment Protocol

Galen (131-201 AD) argues that concentration should be given on the different kinds of foods suitable for blood production rather than on the process of its formation. A person's complexion reflected the presence of thick and thin blood (polycythaemia and anaemia).

Tadeel is one of the principles of treatment of *fasade khūn*. Drugs used for *tadeel* depend upon the nature of *fasad* and involvement of *khilṭ*.

In *hiddate khūn* quantity of blood gets increased, *tadeel* should be done by the use of *tukhme kasni, tukhme kahu, tukhme kishneez, gule surkh, aabe lemu, sikanjaben, sharbate unnab, sharbate sandal, sharbate gajar* etc. provide soothing and cooling effect and ultimately neutralise the *hiddat and ghalayān khūn.*

When *khūn* becomes *raqiq* (decreased viscosity) due to *safrā'*, yellow foam spreads above the blood. Its *tadeel* is done by *mushily safrā'* drugs specially *haleela zard, sharbat unnab, aabe kasni murawwaaq* and those *joshanda* which are used in *ghalba safrā'* and the drugs which are used in *hiddate khūn* can be used in *riqqate khūn.*

If *riqqate khūn* is due to addition of *ghayr tabi'i balgham* colour of blood becomes white. For its *tadeel, mushile balgham* drugs are used. *Haleela kabuli* is very effective. Excessive *rutūbat* of blood can be evacuated by the use of some hot and dry drugs such as *tukhme balanga, tukhme rehan* and *parsiyaunsha.* In this case massage and exercise is also useful.

Ghayr tabi'i ghilzat of blood can be normalised by *sikanjabeen, aabe aalu, aabe badiayn, aabe shahtra and aabe aalu bukhara.* If increase in viscosity is due to *sawdā'* which is most common, blood becomes black and those drugs are effective which are *mukhrije sawdā'* and decreases blood viscosity. If *ghilzat* occurs due to *balgham,* sour drugs and food are beneficial and after *nudj, mushil-i-balgham* drugs are used.

Sometimes blood becomes morbid and putrid. This is the fact that when any *ufūnat* occurs in *khilṭ* fever is compulsory. In this condition cold and dry drugs are beneficial.

Concept of Musaffiyate Khūn Drugs

In *Kitabulfatah* author stated that *mudirre dam* drugs are those which make the blood *lateef* and remove it from the body by opening the pores of vessels. Further the author mentioned that *hareef and murr* drugs clean *fasid* matter and resolve it. In *Al Qanoon Fit Tibb,* Ibn Sina (980-1037AD) used the term *Musaffie khūn.Muqaddama Ilmul advia* it has been mentioned with reference to Jalinoos (AD 131 to 201) that when powder of *Bisfaij* is sprinkled on clotted blood it liquefied the blood, by this observation it was assumed that *bisfaij* has the property of *tasfiya dam.* Hakim Abdul Haleem in *mufradat* compiled a chapter by the name "drugs used in *ahteraq dam*" in which he discussed 52 drugs.

In Unani system of medicine, a lot of single and compound drugs are used to alleviate diverse pathological state caused by *fasade dam.* The single drugs include *unnab, shahtra, mundi, neem, chiraita, chobchini, sarphuka, ushba, sheesham, baram dandi* etc. Several formulations like *arq murakkab mussafie khūn, majone ushba, itrifal shaitra, habbe musaffie khūn, arq musaffie khūn, joshanda musaffie khūn, sharbat unnab, majune musaffie khaas, majune mundi, arq chiraita, arq chob chini* are also used for the same intention. Their detailed description and therapeutic uses has been mentioned in table 1 and 2.

After thorough scrutiny of literature it was noted that all the *musaffie dam* drugs are bitter in taste except *amla, abnus, chob chini* and *unnab.* Most of the drugs are found to be *hārr yābis* in second degree excluding *amla, sandal, mundi* and *unnab.* In general the *quwwate sani* of these drugs are *mulayyin, muhallil, mufattih, mundij, muaddil, jali, ghassal, mujaffif, mulattif, muqatte, muarriq, dāfi'-i-ta'affun* etc. In which some drugs are endowed with the property of *muhallil* viz. *abnus, amla, anjeer dashti, babchi, chiraita, chob chini, neem, panwar, sandal safaid, ushba maghrabi.* Wheares *bakain, barham dandi, chaksu, mundi, panwar, sandal surkh, shahtra* besides *abnus, amla chob chini, sandal safaid,* possess astringent property. On the other hand *neel kanthi, sarphuka, shahtra, ushba maghrabi* together with *abnus, chaksu, chob chini,* possess diuretic activity. Whilst deobstruent is the property of *chiraita, chob chini* and *shahtra,* conversly demulcent activity is confined to *abnus, amla, anjeer dashti, babchi, chiraita, chob chini* and *ushba maghrabi. Abnus* and *shahtra* is desiccant in contrast *Chob chini* and *Ushba* maghrabi have diaphoretic activity. Detergent is the action of *abnus, amla, anjeer dashti, chaksu, shahtra* and *unnab.* By virtue of these properties these drugs act (*quwwate salesa*) as *mushtahi, hādim, muqawwi-i-mi'da wa jigar, mudirr-i-bawl, tiryaq, dāfi'-i-ḥumma, qatile kirme shikam* and *muqawwi-i-a'da' raisa.*

Therapeutic Uses

Generally *musaffie dam* drugs are used in skin diseases and their detailed description is cited in table 1 and 2. However these drugs have some other therapeutic indications which are described below.

According to Ibn Sina (980-1037AD), inspite of hot temperament *abnus* is useful in *harārat khūn;* it arrests hemorrhage if used externally due to its *habis* and *Qabiz* property therefore it is used in *jiryanuddam.* Wheares *amla* prevents *ta'affun* and *fasaad* in *khilṭ* therefore effective in *hiddate khūn as* well due to *qabiz* property it prevents hemaorrhage. Ibn Sina had mentioned in *Advia Qalbiya* that *amla* is beneficial in decreasing *ghilzate khūn,* it helps in production of blood and prevents from premature destruction of blood.At the same time *chobchini* has beneficial role in *su ul qinya* while *chiraita* is found useful in hemorrhage beneath the skin. *Shahtra* is employed in *ihteraqe khūn, ufoonate dam* found very effective in *hiddate khūn, ghilyane khūn* and *hijane khūn.*Some drugs are useful in *ghilzate dam* such as *abnus, amla, babchi, chob chini, shahtra, ushba maghribi* and *bisfaij* while *unnab* is used in *riqqate dam* The temperament of *unnab* is *mu'tadil* and it has the property of *musakkin hiddat khūn, mughallize khūn, mulzije khūn, musaffie khūn, ghasile khūn, tanqiya khūn, munizij akhlāt ghaleeza* and *mushil* by virtue of these properties *unnab* is found very effective in *fasade khūn, hiddat khūn, ghilyan khūn, hijan khūn Panwar* is effective in *surkh bada.* If taken orally for forty days it removes *akhlate fasid* via intestine and purifies blood. *Chob chini* is used in *su ul qinya. Sammul faar mudabbar* in low dose is used as *muqawwi-i-badan* and *musaffie.* Raskapur is also used in fasade *khūn.*

Amla, bakain, barham dandi, neem and *ushba maghrabi* are endowed with the property of *mushile balgham* and used effectively in *balghami* diseases and *balghami* fever. *Chiraita* is used in fever caused by *fasade akhlāt salasa. Sandal safaid* and *sarphuka* cures *safrā'wi* fever. *Shahtra, chiraita, amla, chob chini* and *panwar* remove bad *akhlāt* from body via intestine and reduce fever.

Abnus is used in *sue mizāj māddī* of stomach because it has *mujaffif* and *munaqqi* property by virtue of these actions it removes the morbid matter from stomach. It is also used in malignant abscess. *Chiraita* is used in *waram jigar, warm mi'da* and in digestive problems.

Aabnus, amla, chob chini, sarphuka and *shahtra* are useful in *sawdā'wi* diseases as they remove the morbid *sawdā'* by their *munzij* and *mushile sawdā'* property. *Mundi* is used in *safrā'wi* and *sawdā'wi* diseases and inflammation. *Shahtra* is employed in obstruction of liver and spleen, *sawdā'wi* diseases and jaundice. *Chob chini* acts as *musaffie arwah;* it clears all the morbid humours from the body. *Amla, bakain, barham dandi and neem* and *ushba maghrabi* are endowed with the property of *mushile balgham* and used effectively in *balghami* diseases and fever.[15]

PROPERTIES OF MUSAFFIE DAM DRUGS

Properties	**By and Large**	**Exception**
Taste	Bitter	Sweet/ Pungent
Mizāj / Quwa oola	*Hārr Yābis* in second degree	*Barid yabis/Motadil*
Quwa sani	*jali, mulayyin, muhallil, mufattehe sudad, munzij, muaddil, ghassal, mufattih, mujaffif, mulattif, muqatte, muarriq, dāfi'-i-taffun*	*mubarrid* *musakkin*
Quwa salasa	*muqawwi-i-mi'da* *muqawwi-i-jigar* *mudirr-i-bawl* *mushtahi, hādim* *dāfi'-i-ḥumma* *qatile kirme shikam* *mushily*	*tiryaq* muqawwi-i-a'da' raisa. mushile akhlate salasa muallide dam

Description and Therapeutic Uses of Single Musaffie Dam Drugs

Common name	Scientific name	Parts used	Main therapeutic use/ ailments treated
Abnus	*Diospyros ebenum*	Heart-Wood	Haemorrhage, chronic scabies, *harārate khūn,* flatulence, malignant abscess
Amla	*Emblica officinalis*	Fruit	Fever, heamrorhage, premature destruction of blood, *ghilzat dam*
Anjeer dashti	*Ficus hispida*	Root bark	Leucoderma, blackspot, eczema, warts, pitryasis, dermatophytosis
Babchi	*Psoralea corylifolia*	Seed	*Fasade khūn,* pruritus, pitryasis, leucoderma, melasma/cholasma, ichthyosis, eczema
Barham dandi	*Echinops echinatus*	Leaves	Wound, leucoderma, skin diseases, fasade *khūn,* fasade balgham, chronic fever
Chaksu	*Cassia absus*	Seed Leaves	Vitiligo, wound, leprosy
Chiraita	*Swertia chirata*	Stem leaves	Pupura, hepatitis, gastritis, fever, leprosy, digestive problem pruritus, ringworm, *fasade khūn*

Common name	Scientific name	Parts used	Main therapeutic use/ ailments treated
Chob chini	*Smilax china*	Root	Leprosy, syphilis, wound, ichthyosis, scabies, cancrum, pitryasis, leucoderma, melasma
Mundi	*Sphaera-nthus indicus*	Flower	Ringworm, *safrā'*wi and *sawdā'wi* diseases, inflammation, pruritus, leprosy, boils abscess
Neel kanthi	*Ajuga bracteosa*	Leaves	Erysipelas, pruritus, vitiligo
Neem	*Azadirachta indica*	Flower Fruit Leaves	Boils, abscess, leprosy, pruritus, *safrā'wi* fever, leucoderma, pitryasis, melasma/cholasma
Panwar	*Cassia tora*	Seed	Leprosy, pruritus, melasma, ichthyosis, pityriasis, ring worm
Ras-kapoor	Subchloride of Mercury	Hg_2Cl_2	Syphilis, leprosy, leucoderma
Sammul-far	Arsenic	As	Syphilis, leprosy, leucoderma, pitryasis, malignant wound
Sandal safaid	*Santalum album*	Heart-Wood	Fever, boils and abscess, skin diseases
Sandal surkh	*Pterocarpus santalinus*	Heart-Wood	Urinary tract diseases, skin diseases
Sarphuka	*Tephrosia purpurea*	Whole plant	Boils and abscess, *safrā'*wi wa saudawi fever, *sawdā'wi* diseases

Common name	Scientific name	Parts used	Main therapeutic use/ ailments treated
Shahtra	*Fumaria parviflora*	Whole plant	Scabies, obstruction of liver and spleen, chronic fever, *sawdā'wi* diseases, jaundice, pruritus, Ringworm
Sheesham	*Dalbergia sissoo*	Powder	Leprosy, leucoderma, boils, abscess, *fasade khūn* and *balgham*, syphilis
Unnab	*Zizyphus vulgaris*	Fruit	*Hiddate khūn* pruritus
Ushba	*Smilax aristolochia-efolia*	Root	Syphilis, leprosy, pruritus, melasma/ cholasma, pityriasis, vitiligo

Description and Therapeutic Uses of Compound Musaffie Dam Drugs

Compound drugs	Main ingredient	Therapeutic uses
Arq Mundi	Mundi	*Fasade khūn,* strengthen heart
Arq Murakkab Mussafi Khūn	*Neem, Bakain*	Boils, abscess, syphilis
Arq Shahtra	*Shahtra*	Boils, abscess, *fasade khūn*
Arq Ushba	*Ushba*	*Fasade khūn*
Habbe Daad	*Suhaga-kibreet*	Ringworm
Habbe Kath	*Kath*	Syphilis
Habbe Musaffie Khun	-	*Fasade khūn*
Habbe Qooba	*Seemab, kibreet*	Ringworm
Itrifal Shahtra	*Shahtra*	Pruritus, favus, syphilis
Johar Kala	*Raskapoor*	Syphilis
Majun Chob Chini	*Chob Chini*	*Fasade khūn*
Majun Mundi	*Mundi*	*Fasade khūn*
Majun Musaffie Khas	-	*Fasade khūn,* pruritus
Majun Ushba	*Ushba*	*Fasade khūn,* pruritus
Marham Bars Jadeed	*Babchi*	Vitiligo, pitriyasis, melasma
Marham Kharish Jadeed	*Hina*	Pruritus
Marham Qooba	*Sindoor, safeeda*	Ringworm

Compound drugs	**Main ingredient**	**Therapeutic uses**
Roghan Bars Jadeed	*Babchi*	Vitiligo
Roghan Qooba	*Kameela/ neem*	Ringworm
Sharbat Unnab	*Unnab*	*Ghilzate dam*
Sharbat Murakkab Musaffie Khūn	*Unnab, Haleela*	*Fasade dam*

AABNOOS

Vernaculars		
Arabic	:	Aabnoos
Persian	:	Aabnoos
Hindi	:	Abnus, Ebanus
Marathi	:	Abnus, Karmar
English	:	Indian Ebony
Latin	:	Diospyros ebenum
Syn.	:	Diospyros ebenaster, Diospyros assimilis, Diospyros timoriana
Family	:	Ebenaceae

Introduction and History

Ebony is a dense black hardwood, most commonly yielded by several different species in the genus Diospyros, which also contains the persimmons. It is finely-textured and has a very smooth finish when polished, making it valuable as an ornamental wood. The word ebony comes from the Ancient Egyptian hbny, through the Ancient Greek ἔβενος (ébenos), into Latin and Middle English.

Habit and Habitat:

The tree is found in Orissa, South India, Sri Lanka, Africa and Indonesia.

Description in Unani:

It is a big tree, having oval shaped leaves. Its fruit resembles grapes and are yellowish red in colour. They taste sour and slightly sweet. Seeds and flowers are like of henna plant. Its wood is very heavy and dark black in colour even after breaking it is black from inside also.

Botanical description:

This middle-high evergreen tree grows very slowly up to 20–25 meters (66–82 ft) tall. The leaves are entire-like and have a prolonged oval form, about 6–15 centimeters (2.4–5.9 in) long and 3–5 centimetres (1.2–2.0 in) wide. The fruit is not very big, approximately 2 centimetres (0.79 in) in diameter. It resembles small persimmon fruit. Sap wood is light yellowish gray. The wood core is glossy-black seldom with occasional light fibers. This wood with metallic gloss also has fine and smooth texture. The wood grains can be straight, a bit chaotically organized and wavy. Dry wood density is 1190 kg/m3.

Parts used: wood

Chemical constituents:

Lupeol, Betulin, Betulinic acid, Ursolic acid, Bauerenol, β-sitiosterol, Stigmasterol etc.

Mizaj: Hot dry 2

Pharmacological actions:

Carminative, astringent, laxative, blood purifier, anti inflammatory, demulcent, detergent, aphrodisiac and anti anaemic.Daf-eHiddat-e-Safra (antibilious); Habis (Retentive); Habis-edam (haemostatic), Jali (detergent); Mohallile-Riyah (antiflatulence), Mohallil-e-warm (anti-inflammatory); Mueen-eHamal (conceptive); Mufattit-e-Hisath (lithotriptic); Mufattit-e-Sudad (deobstuent) Mujaffif (desiccant); Mulattifi-e-Mawad (demulscent); Mundamile-Qurooh (wound healer); Muqawwi-e-Basar (tonic for optic nerve); Musaffi-e-Khoon (blood purifier); Musakkin (anxiolytic) Qabiz (astringent); Rade (repellent).

Unani mechanism of action:

Ibne Sina quoted that, Inspite of being hot in temperament a group of Unani physician claimed Abnus reduces the heat of blood. As the one of the action of Abnus is jali because of this action it drains the toxins/impurities from the skin through skin pores hence cleans the imputities. Ibne sina written that jali drugs posses properties of Talien Tabyat which might be another reason for its blood purification properties.

Therapeutic uses:

To treat the snake bite, epiphora (dam-aa), night blindness, weakened eyesight, vascular kereraritis (jaala), diarrhea, biliousness, ulcer, epistaxis, burns, scabies. Harq wa salaq (burn and scald); Hasat-e-kulya (nephrolithisis), Jarb (scabies); Juzam (leprosy); Naar Faarsi (eczema); Nuzool-alMaa (cataract); Qurooh-e-Chashm (wounds of eye); Qurooh-e-Khabisa (chronic wounds); Ratondi (night blindness), Ruaaf (epistaxis); Sailaan-e-Khoon (bleeding); Sailaan-e-mani (spermatorea); Sudad-etihal (spleenic obstruction), Uqr (female sterility); Zof-e-Basar (asthenopia/amblyopia).

Dose: 5-7 gms

Mode of Use:

Powder of its wood is usually used in eye diseases. It is sprinkled on wounds locally. It is used as surma (kohl).

Research Studies:

Antifungal activity, Antioxidant, Antibacterial activity

Toxicity: Toxic to stomach, hepatic disorder.

Corrective: Honey

Substitutes: Burada Sheesham

Compound formulations: Sharbat Murakkab Musaffie khun

AFTEEMOON

Vernaculars		
Persian	:	Darakht e pechan
Hindi	:	Aakash bel
Gujrati	:	Amar bel
Marathi	:	Aakas vel
English	:	Dodder, love vine
Latin	:	Cuscuta reflexa, Roxb
Family	:	Convolvulaceae
Mizaj	:	Afteemoon : Hot^2 Dry^2, Tukhm e kashoos : Hot^1 Dry^2
Part used	:	vine, seeds

Introduction and History

Cuscuta seeds have long been used for osteoporosis in China and some other Asian countries. Cuscuta is a commonly used traditional Chinese medicine which is believed to strengthen the liver and kidney.

Habit and Habitat:

It is found at the temperate and tropical regions of the world with huge species diversity in tropical and subtropical regions.It is common throughout India(U.P., Punjab, Bengal, South Indian region), abundant in Bengal plains. About 6 species are found in India.

Botanical description:

Cuscuta reflexa Roxb. Is a rootless, leafless perennial parasitic twining herb of Convolvulaceae family, commonly known as Akashvalli or Dodder. It has no chlorophyll and cannot make its own food by photosynthesis. It grows on thorny or other shrubs, sometimes completely covering the bushes and trees. it spreads from one host to another, and on each victim, they twine and cling tightly with special branching organs called haustorium. Haustorium penetrate the host and connect to the host xylem as well as to the host phloem and absorbs from it both water and elaborated food stuffs such as sugar and amino acids. It lives its entire life without attachment to the ground and grows with the help of seeds which are minute and produced in large quantities. Seeds have hard coating, and survive in the soil for 5-10 yrs or more. It varies in the colour of flowers produced from white to pink.

Unani description:

It's a parasitic plant which grows on stems of other trees. It resembles fine thread of golden yellow colour. Summer and spring are favorable seasons for its spread. Flowers are bell shaped and of multiple colours, can be white, yellow or blue. Fruits are formed from flower, inside the fruit; small grayish yellow seeds are present which are called 'Tukhm e kashoos'. According to the place where cuscuta is seen, it is of 2 types. (1) Afteemoon Vilayati and (2) Afteemoon Hindi. Afteemoon vilayati is comparatively thin and more potent in function.

Pharmacological Actions:

Hepatoprotective, Anti-flatulant, Digestive, Expels saudawi akhlat, Antipyretic, Anti-inflammatory, Blood purifier, Stomach tonic, deobstruent, diuretic, emenogogue, demulcent, laxative, analgesic, concative, etc.

Unani mechanism of action:

Afteemon is a drug of choice for saudawi disbalance. It cleans the impure sawda in blood by expelling excessive or disbalance sawdawi khilt. The primary action or taseer oola is demulcent and anti inflammatory which also leads to blood cleansing action.

Therapeutic Uses:

Used in saudawi diseases like *junoon, maalenkhulia, kaaboos.* Disturbed function of liver, stomach and spleen, indigestion, jaundice, intestinal worms, blood disorders and chronic fever. It is locally applicable on wound and promotes healing and alopecia.

Chemical constituents:

Cuscutin, quercetin, amarbelin, amino acids, cuscutaline, scoparone, melanettin, hyperoside, aromadendrin, taxifolin, astragalin, myricetin, kaempferol, apigenin 7-O- glucoside, luteolin, quercetin, 6,7 – dimethoxy -2H-1 benzopyran -2-one, 3-(3,4- dihydroxyphenyl) -2- propen- 1- ethanoate, 6,7,8- trimethoxy- 2H- benzopyran- 2- one, 3-(4- O- β- D- glucopyranoside- 3,5- dimethoxyphenyl)- 2- propen- 1 –ol β- sitosterol, α- amyrin, β- amyrin, β- amyrin acetate, α- amyrin acetate, oleanolic acetate, oleanolic acetate, oleanolic acid, lupeol, 3β- hydroxyolean- 12(13)- enetridecanoate and heptadecanoate, coumarin, 3,4-O- dicaffeoylquinic acid, 3-Ocaffeoylquinic acid, D- mannitol, myricetin 3- O- α- rhamnoside.

Mode of Use:

Application of crushed and boiled Akashbel on fistula helps in healing.In splenomegaly local application is very effective. Steam of decoction relieves pain.

Drinking with vinegar relieves hiccups. Infusion is effective in jaundice.

Research studies:

Hypotensive and bradycardiac effects, Antidiabetic effect, Antioxidant activity, Antipyretic activity, Spasmolytic action, Anti-HIV activity, Antitumor activity, Anti-arthritic and nephroprotective effect, Anti-inflammatory activity, Antimicrobial activity, Hair growth activity, Relaxant and spasmolytic action, Cholinergic action, Antistredogenic activity, Hepatoprotective activity, Hypoglycemic activity, Anticonvulsant activity,

Dose : 3-5 gm

Toxicity : Toxic to lungs

Correctives: Kaasni (Chicory), Sikanjabeen

Substitute: Afsanteen (Artemisia absinthium)

Compound formulations: Maajoon e najah, Maajoon e ushba, Sharbate deenar, Maajoon e dabidulward, Itrifal afteemoon.

AMLA

Vernaculars		
Arabic	:	Amlaj
Persian	:	Aamla
Urdu	:	Anwala, Aamla, Amlika
Hindi	:	Amalak, Amvala, Amlika, Anwla
English	:	Emblic myrobalan, Indian gooseberry
Latin	:	*Emblica officinalis* Gaertn.
Syn.	:	*Phyllanthus emblica* Linn.
Family	:	Euphorbiaceae

Introduction and History

Amla fruit is used since ancient times for the treatment of various ailments.

Habit and Habitat:

It's a medium size tree of 10 to 15 meter high. It is found wildly and also cultivated in all parts of India, especially in south, to an altitude of 1500 m, the Deccan, sea cost districts and Kashmir. Although it is native to India, also grows in tropical and subtropical regions of Pakistan, Uzbekistan, Srilanka, South East Asia, China and Malaysia. In India it is cultivated in UP, MP, Tamil Nadu and Rajasthan.

Description in Unani:

The bark of tree is light brownish in color. Leaves are compound; its upper surface is light green while lower surface is more pallor which emit lemon odour. Flowers are yellowish white and fruits are globular in shape of a diameter of 2.5-3.5 cm, but the fruit obtained from cultivated plants are bigger in size sometimes reached up to 8 cm in diameter. Fruits are pulpy and divided into 6 lobes by white lines. Its seeds are also divided by ridges. Unripe fruit is green, half ripe fruit is yellowish and after complete ripening it becomes reddish brown. Dried fruits are wrinkled. The taste of fruit is sour and astringent. A type is described by Unani physicians which are not sour or astringent in taste and shape is slightly flat that is called as *Shah amla* or *Amlajul mulook* or *Shalghami amla*. The average weight of a fruit is 60-70 gm.

Botanical description:

It is a small medium sized deciduous tree with smooth, greenish grey, exfoliating bark. Leaves are feathery with small narrowly oblong, pinnately arranged leaflets. Fruits are depressed globose ½ - 1 inch in diameter, fleshy and obscurely 6-lobed, containing 6 small seeds. The tree is 30-40 ft in height and circumference of stem usually extends up to 3-6 ft and rarely up to 9 ft. Stem is usually curved, branches are strong and extended. Bark is thin and brownish in colour. Leaves resemble to tamarind leaves. Fruits are fleshy and round in shape. Raw fruits are green in colour and become greenish yellow on ripening. Fruit contain a three celled nut each cell of which contain two triangular seeds. Seeds are round, edges of which are sharp.

Parts used: Fruit and Roghan amla

Chemical constituents:

Amla is a good source of vitamin C. One kg of fresh amla contains 6000 unit of vit. C and 500 calories. It also has calcium, phosphorus and iron content. Quercetin, phyllaemblic compounds, gallic acid, tannins, flavonoids, pectin and glucose are also reported in amla fruit. On long storage, its tannin and vit. c contents got reduced therefore it is better if used within 2 years. Dried fruit contains more amount of gallic acid.

Mizaj: Cold[1], Dry[2]

Pharmacological actions:

Stomach tonic, liver tonic, tonic to vital organs, anti diarrheal, astringent, blood purifier, appetizer, detergent, anti inflammatory, phlemagogue, melanogogue, decreases the elevated heat of blood. According to Shaikh and Gilani amla decreases *hararat* and *safrawyat* of *khoon,* prevent *akhlat* from *taffun* and *fasad,* strengthens the eyesight, strengthens the root of hair as well as darkens thems.

Unani mechanism of action:

Amla reduces the heat. It maintains the temperament of blood due to its *musaffie dam* property. According to Avicenna as mentioned in advia *qalbiya* that amla is beneficial in decreasing the viscosity of blood, less production of blood and in premature destruction of blood. Tone ups the stomach, intestine, liver and heart due to its astringent property. It strengthens the stomach enabling it for better coction, relieves thirst, stop vomiting and improve appetite. It prevents the drainage of matter to the lower part of the body that is why it is found very effective in piles and *zalqul ama.* It also dries the excessive fluid of brain and provides strength and increases intellect. Amla effectively expels the excessive *balghami* and *saudawi mawad* from the body. When the blood is purified from these filthy matters, *roohe haiwani* and *roohe nafsani* are ultimately purified resulting in strengthening of heart and brain. It strengthens the root of hair due to its astringent property. Since it dries the excessive fluid that's why it is very useful in strengthening the nerves. It delays the aging process. Ibn Sina says that amla is better than halela as it dries cold phlegmatic fluid from the body.

Therapeutic uses:

Used in *Saudawi* disease, To prevent hemorrhage, weakness of liver, stomach and heart, to improve the memory power and sharpens the eyesigh, *hiddate safra wa khoon,* in relieving thirst and to control diarrhea.Its extract is applied or used as a wash to strengthen the eyesight.Its decoction is used to wash the hair in premature graying of the hair, falling of hair. It is used as an ingredient in hair dyes and shampoos.

Dose: 3-5gm; 7gm; 10.5 gm

Mode of Use:

Amla is very astringent in nature so always *Amla sheer parwarda* is used which is prepared by soaking in milk.

Its powder is mixed with equal quantity of sugar and a little amount of almond oil. This recipe is very effective in weakness of eyesight if it is consumed in the dose of 15 gm.

Amla powder in the dose of 7 gm is used to normalise the excessive heat of blood caused by safra (*hiddate safra wa khoon*)

Amla is soaked in water for a while the same water if consumed very effective in relieving thirst.

Habbe amla and its infusion are very effective in diarrhea and thirst.

Murabba amla wrapped with waraqe nuqra is used in palpitation and weakness of brain.

Sharbate amla is considered best in all the preparations. Sharbate amla with lemon juice is used in acute bacillary dysentery.

If amla is used as a toffee, effective in excessive salivation and strengthens the gums.

Amla with balchar is the best remedy to strengthen the stomach and intestine.

It is used with iron in anemia, jaundice and dyspepsia

Roghan amla is used to strengthen the hair and brain.

Research Studies

A lot of research studies have been carried out on this drug

Amla is found effective in hyperchlorhydria; it has antidyspeptic activity

Amla is effective in gastric ulcer; it's both gastro protective and anti secretory activities has been reported.

Amla is hepatoprotective.

Its anti inflammatory, antipyretic and spasmolytic activity has been recorded.

Amla is found effective against large number of bacteria and viruses.

It also has cytoprotective and antioxidant activity.

Toxicity: Toxic to spleen, may cause constipation and colitis.

Correctives: Honey and Almond oil

Substitute: For stomach halela siyah, and Kabuli.

Compound formulations:

Jawarishe Amla, Murabbae Amla, Anushdaru, Safoofe hazim Itrifalat, Dawawul misk motadil sada

ANJEER DASHTI

Vernaculars		
Arabic	:	Teen barri
Persian	:	Anjir Dashti
Urdu	:	Jangli Anjeer
Hindi	:	Kathomri, gobla, kala umbar, katgularia, phalgu
English	:	Wild fig, hairy fig, opposite-leaved fig-tree, rough-leaved fig tree
Latin	:	*Ficus hispida* Linn. Syn. *Covellia hispida* (Linnaeus f.) Mique
Family	:	Moraceae

Introduction and History

In India the use of Anjeer dates back to the time of Charaka when he advised the juice obtained from the fig to be taken with jaggery as a mild purgative in the treatment of vitiligo. The fruit juices along with honey act as a good antihemorrhagic. It has been cultivated for over 11,000 years._*Ficus hispida* is a valuable plant due to its various pharmacological activities. *Ficus hispida* derived from the Latin word FIK-us "for Fig" and HISS-pih- duh means "with bristly hairs".

Habit and Habitat:

Ficus hispida is a shrub or moderate sized tree, found throughout the year, growing in evergreen forest, moist localities, banks of stream, deciduous forests, to an elevation of 1800 m above sea level, often cultivated in villages for shade and its edible fruits in India, Sri Lanka, Myanmar, southern region of the Republic of China, New Guinea, Australia and Andaman Island. In India mostly found in Punjab, Bengal and Rajasthan

Description in Unani:

Ficus hispida is a medium sized and very fast growing tree. Fruitining takes place within two or three years. Flowers and fruits remain throughout the year. Its leaves are rough and 4-12 inches long with oval shape but inferior surface is covered with minute hair. The leaves are arranged in opposite manner. Its fruits are triangular, one inch long and found in a group of two. Its fruits are similar as anjeer Bustani but small in size. Unripe fruits are green, then yellowish green but after complete ripening its looks like the colour of jamun. Taste is sweet and used in making jam. A type of milky secretion oozes after breaking of any part of this tree which has some sticky gum like properties. Hakim Najmul Ghani has described its three varieties small, large and spiny.

Botanical description:

It is a coarsely hairy shrub or medium sized tree, up to 10 m tall. Bark is generally brownish or blaze pink. Leaves are simple, decussate, ovate, oblong, or obovate-oblong, thickly papery, covered with coarse hairs and oppositely arranged on 1–4 cm long petiole; margin is entire or dentate, sometimes irregularly toothed. Inflorescence is of syconia type, clustered on tubercles of main trunk, older branches and sometimes on pendulous leafless branches. Male flowers are many and found near apical pore; calyx is three lobed, thinly membranous; stamen 1. Gall flowers: calyx is absent; style subapical, short, and thick. Female flowers: calyx lobes absent; style lateral with hairs appearing during the months of June and July. Figs appear in leaf axil on normal leafy shoots, sometimes on leafless branchlets, solitary or paired, yellow or red when mature, top-shaped and 1.2–3 cm in diameter.

Parts used: Root bark, Fruit, leaves

Chemical constituents:

Preliminary phytochemical investigations have shown the presence of alkaloids, carbohydrates, proteins and amino acids, sterols, phenols, flavonoids, gums and mucilage, glycosides, saponins, and terpenes. It also possesses phenanthroindolizidine alkaloids, n-alkanes, coumarins and triterpenoids. Leaves of the plant contain hispidin, oleanolic acid, bergapten, β-amyrin and β-sitosterol. Bark comprises of lupeol acetate, β-sitosterol and β-amyrin acetate. Ficustriol and phenanthroindolizidine alkaloid Omethylthylophorindine has also been isolated from this plant.

Mizaj: Hot and Dry. It is potent than *Ficus carica*

Pharmacological actions:

Musaffie khoon, muhammir, Qawi muhallil, qawi muharriq, qawi detergent, qawi mushil, mulattif

Unani mechanism of action:

Anjeer Dashti is more hot and toxic and stronger in all the actions than Anjeer Bustani. It is characterized by hirreef and yabis a property that's why it is *qawi mulattif, muqatte* and *mushil*. By virtue of these actions it purifies blood from excessive viscid *balghami* and *saudawi rutoobat* through ishal and cure leucoderma and other skin diseases when used orally. Further due to its *jali, muhammir, mukharrish* and *muharriq* property its *zemad* is applied in ring worm, leucoderma, Melasma, cholasma and wart.

Therapeutic uses:

On the basis of above pharmacological actions the drug is usually used in skin diseases such as warts, pityriasis, blemishes, ring worm, leucoderma, dark spots and eczema.

Dose: Root bark 2-5gm

Mode of Use:

Unripe anjeer fruit if used as a dusting powder or its paste is applied with vinegar and salt on scalp very effective in the ulcers of scalp.

The *zemad* of ripened anjeer is effective in cervical lymphadenitis.

Its root either used orally or as liniment is considered best remedy for epilepsy.

Its milk is applied on freckles, wart and ring worm

Its root bark is used with vinegar as liniment in ring worm.

In leucoderma its root bark powder is used orally in the dose of 500 mg and externally it is applied on affected parts after grinding in rose water and continues to use for 40 days.

The paste of unripe fruit alone or with vinegar and salt is applied on scalp to cure baldness.

Powdered unripe fruits used as a zemad on vitiligo as it possess a definite photosensitizing activity.

Research Studies:

A lot of research studies have been carried out on this drug especially on leaves.

The methanol soluble fraction, crude ethanol extract and n-hexane soluble fraction of various parts of *F. hispida* showed thrombolytic activity.The hepatoprotective effect of methanolic extract of leaves is reported against cyclophosphamide mediated oxidative liver injury in Wistar rat. Hepatoprotective activity of leaves extract against paracetamol induced acute liver damage in rats is also reported.Water-soluble portion of the ethanol extract of *Anjeer dashti* showed hhypoglycaemic activity. The cardioprotective effect of leaf extract on cyclophosphamide mediated myocardial injury due to oxidative stress in rat heart is demonstrated.The methanolic extract of leaves showed a significant antidiarrheal activity. The methanolic extract of root in aspirin ulcerated rats showed decreased the incidence of ulcers, enhanced the healing of ulcers and significantly reduced free and total acidity.The methanolic extract of leaves has ssedative and anticonvulsant effects.The neuroprotective effect of methanolic extract of leaves on b-amyloid induced cognitive deficits and oxidative stress in mice is reported.Ethanolic fraction is found to have anti-neoplastic activity against T47D cells. Its leaves exhibited antitumor activity. Leaves extract has anti-inflammatory and antipyretic effect.

Toxicity: emetic

Correctives: Sikanjbeen

Substitute: For vitiligo babchi

Compound formulations: Zimaad kibreet, Safufe bars

Babchi

Vernaculars

Arabic	:	Mahhlab aswad
Urdu	:	Babchi, Babechi, Bakuchi, Bavachi
Hindi	:	Babachi, Babchi, Bavanchiyan, Bakuci
English	:	Babchi seeds, *Psoralea* seeds, Malay tea, Scurf-pea, Fountain bush
Latin	:	*Psoralea corylifolia* Linn.
Family	:	Fabaceae

Introduction and History

Babchi has an immense biological importance and it has been widely exploited since ages for its magical effect against several skin diseases such as psoriasis, leucoderma and leprosy. But Arab physicians were not aware about this plant. It was included in Unani medicine in 18 th century. Its medicinal uses have been mentioned in Indian pharmaceutical codex, the Chinese, British and American Pharmacopoeas. The most amazing aspect of this plant is that every part is useful in skin diseases. It is also called as Kushthanashini (leprosy destroyer).

Habit and Habitat:

Psoralea corylifolia is an annual herb. It is actually a winter season weed and grows throughout the plains of India, especially in the semi-arid regions of Rajasthan and Eastern districts of Punjab, adjoining Uttar Pradesh. It is also found throughout India in Himalayas, Dehra Dun, Bundelkhand, Bengal, and Bombay, some valley in Bihar, Deccan, and Karnataka. This plant is also widely distributed in the tropical and subtropical regions of the world, especially China and Southern Africa.

Description in Unani:

The plant of Babchi is an annual, erect herb; 30-180 cm high. Its flowers are yellowish or bluish in colour; leaves are small and somewhat rounded. It has elongated pods which are dark brown or black containing black seed. It has no odour; after chewing gives pungent taste.

Botanical description:

Seeds are brownish black in colour, oblong, and flattened or kidney shaped, 2–4 mm long, 2–3 mm broad, and 1–1.5 mm thick, hard, smooth, exalbuminous with straw-colored testa, with an agreeable aromatic odour and a pungent-bitter taste. They have grooved and gland-dotted stems. Leaves are simple, broadly elliptic, rounded, and mucronate at apex, clothed with white hairs on both surfaces, covered with numerous black dots, 5 main nerves springing from the base. Flowers are dense, corolla yellow or bluish purple, axillary, 10–30 flowered racemes. Flowering time is from August to December. Fruit is small, 5 mm long, subglobular, slightly compressed, pitted black, beaked without hairs, indehiscent, one-seeded pod, which is adhering to the pericarp.

Parts used: Seeds, seed oil, roots and leaves.

Chemical constituents: Seeds contain volatile oil 0.05%, brown fixed oil 10 %, and dark brown resin 8.6%, a pigment hydroxyflavone. The seed and roots contain chalcones, flavones, isoflavones, furanocoumarins and coumesterol group of compounds. It also has flavonoids such as bavachin, bavachinin and corylin. Coumarin contents include psoralen, isopsoralen, psoraledin and angelicin.

Mizaj: Hot and dry in second or third degree

Pharmacological actions:

Externally it is *jali, mukharrash* and *muhammire jild*

Internally it is *mulattif, muhallil, mushile balgham* and *musaffie khoon.*

Unani mechanism of action:

Babchi due to its *mulattif* and *mushil balgham* property expelles the abnormal phlegmatic matter from the body and purify the blood.

Therapeutic uses:

fasade khoon, pruritus, pitryasis, leucoderma, melasma/cholasma, ichthyosis, eczema, fasade badan, black spot, leprosy, skin diseases.

Dermatitis and other edematous condition of skin such as boils and skin eruptions.

Scorpion sting and snake bite.

Dose: Powder 3.5 to10 gm, infusion 15 gm

Mode of Use:

Its powder is used internally and a paste is made with powder applied on the affected area.

Babchi, gulnar, geru and sulphar are taken in equal amount and soaked in water overnight; in morning its decanted water is taken orally and the remaining part is used as paste on the affected area.

Research Studies

Oleo resinous extract of seeds are found more effective in leucoderma.Mixture of psoralen and isopsoralen if used orally also produce good results.When used locally in leucoderma it dilate the vessels and plasma increased to that area and skin becomes red and melanoblast stimulated because its function is disturbed in vitiligo, babchi stimulate and leads to them to form and exudates pigments which gradually diffuses into white patches.Alcoholic extract of the seeds reported for anthelmintic, anti viral and antibacterial activities.Seed powder and extract contain corylin, corylifolin, bakuchiol and psoraliacin which have antioxidant activity.It also has anti inflammatory and anti tumour activity. Seed extract has protective effects on oxidative stress and mitochondrial function in hepatocytes.Antifungal activity of petroleum ether extract of seedS reported against *Fusarium* species.Effects of seed extract on beta cell death were seen. Oral administration of extract resulted in a significant improvement of hyperglycemia, glucose tolerance and increased serum insulin levels in streptozotocin-induced diabetic mice.Hexane and chloroform fractions showed estrogenic activity in yeast trans activation assay and E. screen assay.Bavachinin, corylifolinin, and psoralen inhibit the multiplication of osteosarcoma and lung cancer cells. They are also useful in fibrosarcoma, malignant ascites, and leukemia.The total furanocoumarins present in babchi possess potent and rapid antidepressant properties that are mediated via MAO, the hypothalamic–pituitary–adrenal axis, Its Immuno modulatory activity has also been reported.

Toxicity:

Prolong oral use may cause nausea, vomiting and headache and sometimes may cause diarrhea due to GIT irritation.

Excessive exposure of ultraviolet light increases excessive bile secretion and acute cholestatic hepatic injury, therefore it should not be given in patients suffering of liver diseases, lupus erythematosus, hydroaporphyria and other diseases associated with light sensitivity.

Studies discovered that psoralen cause reproductive toxicity

Correctives: Sikanjabeen and other tursh drugs

Substitute: Suddab, atrilal

Compound formulations: Sufoof bars, zemad bars

Bakain

Vernaculars

Arabic	:	Alzanz lakht
Persian	:	Azad darakht
Urdu	:	Mahanim
Hindi	:	Bakai, bakain,
English	:	Cape lilac, indian or persian lilac, white cedar
Latin	:	*Melia azedarach* Linn.,
Syn.	:	*Melia composita* Willd., *Melia dubia* Cavanilles, *Melia japonica* Don.
Family	:	Meliaceae

Introduction and History

The whole plant or specific parts (leaves, stem, and roots) of bakain are known to have medicinal properties and have a long history of use by indigenous and tribal people in India.

Habit and Habitat:

Melia azedarach is a small to medium deciduous tree attaining a height up to 45 m; bole fluted below when old, up to 30-60 (max. 120) cm in diameter, with a spreading crown and sparsely branched limbs. It is grown as an ornamental avenue tree and sometimes as a shade tree in coffee and tea plantation. The tree is hardy and draught resistant and is found grown widely in the sub Himalayan region up to 2000 m above sea level.

Description in Unani:

Bakain is a large well known tree found in most of the parts of India. It was introduced in India by Persian physicians since then its cultivation was started. It is more or less similar to neem that's why it is also called as vilayeti neem. Its length may go upto 40 feet. Stem is erect and leaves are similar to neem but small in size and soft. Flowers are aromatic, blakish white with reddish tinge; Fruits are yellow, inside the fruits there are 4-5 seeds. Rind of seed is black which has bitter and pungent taste and little amount of fixed oil which is similar to neem oil. A blue colour is obtained by boiling its leaves. All parts of the plant are bitter in taste similar to neem with same pharmacological properties.

Botanical description:

Leaves are two to three-times compound, alternate and pubescent to glabrous. Leaflets are 2-8 cm long, serrate or crenate, dark green above, often with sparse hairs along the veins and lighter green and generally smooth below. The inflorescence is a panicle from leaf axils and form leafless nodes on the lower part of the new growth. Sepals are green, 1.5-2 mm long. Petals are pinkish lavender, ligulate, 1-1.3 cm long. Stamens are united into a cylindrical, dark purple tube, 6-8 mm long and cut at the apex into 15-25 slender teeth. Flowers are fragrant. The fruit is a stalked, one seeded drupe that is greenish yellow to yellowish tan, globose and 1-1.5 cm in diameter.

Parts used: Leaves, root bark, fruit

Chemical constituents

Root bark contains resinous matter. The rind of its seed has some bitter substances. Root contains some active constituents viz. bakainin, melianin, nimbinie, azaridin, meliacin, quercetin, rutin, margosin, kaempferol, lupeol, beta sitosterol, sugar and tannin.

Mizaj: hot ^{2} dry ^{2}

Pharmacological actions:

Leaves: *muhallile awram, musaffie khoon*

Root bark: *Qatile kirm shikam, dafe taffun*

Fruit: *Musakkine dard, mulain, mudirre haiz*

Unani mechanism of action:

Its flowers are exhilarant and strengthen the heart and brain, effective in chronic headache. Seeds are useful in expelling of viscous humour and relieve obstruction if used with water. All parts of the plant have *jila* and *taqtee* property by virtue of this effective in barsh, namash, kalaf, bahaq and qurooh and fade up the blakish spots. Its fruits expel the phlegmatic matter through purgation. The buds remove obstructions from brain.

Therapeutic uses:

Its leaves and root bark is used in diseases caused by fasade khoon, boils, abscess, leprosy and chronic *balghami* fever. Its roghan is used in diseases caused by *sauda*

Dose: Root bark 7gm to 10 gm, fruit 0.5 to 1 gm.

Mode of Use:

Fresh juice of its leaves or decoction is used in all the diseases.

A warm paste is prepared from its leaves and applied on the glandular swellings.

An ointment is prepared from its leaves and used in skin diseases.

Vapor of leaves decoction is used to reduce pain.

Decoction of root bark is used orally several times at an interval of three hours in worm infestation.

Its two seeds are soaked in water then ground and use with honey in worm infestation.

Decoction of its bark mixed with the juice of fumitory and myrobalan processed by the method of *tarweeq* is useful in phlegmatic fever.

Research Studies

Seeds are found effective in gastric and duodenal ulcers.Leaves have immuno modulatory properties.Leaves and fruits have anti feedent properties.Meliacin is found in the leaves has anti viral activity against herpes simplex.The whole plant has anti fungal, anti bacterial, anti malarial and anthelmintic activities.The whole plant has insecticidal and rodenticidal activities.It's analgesic and anti inflammatory activity has also been demonstrated.The whole plant has antifertility and antilithiatic activity.It also has Cytotoxic and antiproliferative activity.

Toxicity: The fruit is sometimes poisonous, toxic to stomach and liver and causes pain even lethal for chest

Corrective: Anisoon

Substitutes: Majeeth in equal quantitiy, taj in half quantity and javitri in one tenth parts

Compound formulations: Habbe bawaseer, Majoon Musakkine dard reham

Barham Dandi

Vernaculars		
Urdu	:	*Barham dandi, Labh, Untkatara, Jachir*
Hindi	:	*Gokhru, Uthkanta, Utakatira*
English	:	Indian globe thistle, Camel's thistle, yellow thistle
Latin	:	*Tricholepis chaetolepis* (Boiss.) Rech. f. *Echinops echinatus* Roxb.
Family	:	Asteraceae

Introduction and History

The drug "Barham Dandi", botanically the Tricholepis chaetolepis (Bioss). Rech. f. of family Asteraceae occupies a pivotal role in the Unani, Ayurvedic and indigenous system of medicine since long. The aerial parts are known for their therapeutic and pharmaceutical properties such as antipyretic, nerve tonic and skin infections. There are number morphologically closely related specie of family Asteraceae are traded throughout the world for same pharmaceutical. However, two most widely used and traded species instead of *T. chaetolepis* includes *Oligochaeta ramosa* (Roxb.) Wagenitz and *Acroptilon repens* (L.) DC. are also known as Barham Dandi. It is interesting to note that these two drugs have quite different pharmaceutical application than *T. chaetolepis.*

This drug is also confused in classical Unani literature such as Mohite Azam, Yadgar Razai, Makhzanul Advia, Makhzanul Mufradat. This drug is usually referred to by their vernacular names. As a result, the botanical identity of this plant has remained doubtful even today in common practices by markets and herbal industries. The name Barham Dandi is attributed to more than one plant species such as *Argemone maxicana, T. chaetolepis, Lamprachaenium microaphalatum, Echinops echinatus,* and *Echinops glabbariana.*

Habit and Habitat

It is widely distributed in the desert regions of Africa, the Mediterranean, India, and the Southeast Asian countries. Its root, leaves, fruit, and bark are the most commonly used parts. Within India, it grows at an altitude of 1,500 m throughout the country. It is ordinarily present on and along roadsides, grasslands, and open forest areas.

Description in Unani:

It is an herb found all over India. It is an annual plant of 20-60 cm. in height. Branches are thin and green. Flowers are reddish blue in colour. Its every part is spiny. All parts of this plant are bitter in taste but leaves are more bitter.

Botanical description:

A rigid, pubescent, annual herb up to 1-3 ft height, with branches widely spreading from the base. **Leaves** alternate, sessile, oblong, pinnatifid, covered with cottony wool beneath, the lobes triangular and oblong, simuate and spiny, the spines often 2.5 cm long, deeply pinnatifid, leaves are 7-12 cm long. **Flower** heads white or purple, compact, globose, clustered at the ends of branches; involucres surrounded by strong white bristles resembling pappus-hairs; pappus short, yellowish, forming a short cylindrical brush above the achene. Heads occur in solitary white spherical balls, 3-5 cm across.

Parts used: Whole plant

Chemical constituents:

TLC of aerial parts extract reveals the presence of smaller amount of flavonol, two minor amounts of phenolic acids and one aurone when viewed under 366 nm UV light.

Mizaj: Hot and dry

Pharmacological actions:

Dafe humma, Dafe humma muzmina, musaffe dam, Muharrike kabid, mudirre safra, mudirre haiz, qatile kirme shikam, tonic, nervine tonic and *Qabiz.*

Unani mechanism of action:

As its taste is bitter and temperament is hot therefore it has a number of pharmacological properties viz. liver tonic, resolvent, deobstruent, diuretic etc. By virtue of these characteristics it is able to transform the morbid viscous matter into such a form which can be easily evacuated by the body.

Therapeutic uses:

Barham dandi is used in all types of fever particularly malarial fever, hepatitis and jaundice, amenorrhoea and intestinal worm, zofe aam, zofe dimagh, jiryan and seelan, skin diseases caused by blood impurities.

Dose: 5-7 gm

Mode of Use:

Its decoction or infusion with other drugs is used in chronic fevers.

Its infusion is used as blood purifier.

If 10 gm is used with cow milk it clears voice, increases intellect, reduces cough and dryness of mouth.

Powder of aerial parts ½ tea spoon thrice a day for 15 days is recommended to treat scabies, skin grains and for other blood impurities.

250 mg powder is taken twice a day with cow milk for fever and mental weakness.

Research Studies:

A lot of research studies have been carried out on this drug.

Analgesic activity:

The methanolic extract of the aerial parts and roots at 250 and 500 mg/kg exhibits significant analgesic activity against hot plate, tail immersion, and tail flick models; it was reported that the methanolic extract

Diuretic activity:

The methanolic extract of the aerial parts and roots showed diuretic activity in an *in vivo* Lipschitz test model. The results show a significant increase in urine volume and electrolyte excretion at 250 mg/kg and 500 mg/kg body weight.

Effect on reproductive organs:

The terpenoid fraction from the petroleum ether extract of the roots at 30 and 60 mg/kg shows a significant decrease in the weight of the reproductive organs. In addition, there was a significant decrease in the levels of serum testosterone and cauda epididymal sperm concentration.

Hepatoprotective activity:

The ethanolic extract at 500 and 750 mg/kg/day has been tested in CCl_4 -intoxicated rabbits for 7 days. The extract shows significant reinstatement in SGPT, SGOT, ALP levels as compared to CCl_4 and Silymarin control groups.

Antioxidant activity:

The free radical-scavenging activity reported in various *in vitro* models, such as the scavenging of 2, 2 diphenyl-1-picrylhydrazyl (DPPH) radical, nitric oxide radical, and superoxide anion.

Anti-inflammatory activity:

The ethanol extract of the whole plant was studied in carrageenan-, formaldehyde- and adjuvant-induced inflammation in rats.

Protective effect on prostate

The butanolic fraction of the ethanolic extract reported for its protective effect on the prostate.

Anti-irritant activity:

The anti-irritant activity in several fractions of the chloroform extract of powdered plant was tested on abraded and irritated rabbit skin. Out of five fractions, two were reported to have significant effect.

Antibacterial activity:

A mother tincture shows antibacterial activity against several microorganisms highly effective against *Salmonella typhi*, moderately effective against *Escherichia coli*, and not very effective against *Pseudomonas aeruginosa* at 200 μg/mL and 400 μg/mL strength of mother tincture.

Antipyretic activity:

The antipyretic activity of the ethanolic extract at 500 mg/kg and 750 mg/kg shows antipyretic activity in rabbit.

Wound-healing activity:

Extracts of *E. echinatus* in petroleum ether, chloroform, ethanol, and distilled water showed wound-healing activity in excision, incision, and dead space wound models.

Toxicity: Causes dryness

Correctives: Honey

Substitute: Mundi and Nil kanth

Compound formulations: Arq Murakkab Musaffie khun banushka khas, sharbat musaffie khun

CHAKSU

Vernaculars

Arabic	:	Shishm, Tashmeezaj
Persian	:	Chashkhaam, Chashmeezak
Urdu	:	Chaksu
Hindi	:	Bankulthi, Chaksu
Ayurvedic	:	Shimbi Kul
English	:	Absus Seeds
Latin	:	Cassia absus Linn
Family	:	Fabaceae

Introduction and History

The important seed of Unani medicine particularly used for Vitiligo since many years

Habit and Habitat: It is mainly distributed in India and Sri Lanka in wastelands up to 1500 m. It is present in all tropical regions across the world

Description in Unani:

Size of the plant is approximately 1 to 3 feet. Stem is thin. Leaves are 1 to 2 inch long green in colour, flower is yellowish small and pod is 1 to 2 feet. Each pod contains 5 to 6 seeds. Seed are triangular in shape, small, shiny, black similar to *bahdana* seed. Seed is purified with Rose water.

Botanical description:

The herbs is 1.2 m in height, Leaves compound, paripinate, leaflets 3-pairs. Flowers are bright yellow, usually in pairs, axillary. Pods are long, slender, obliquely sepatate, 15-25 cm long. Seeds are about 4-4.5 mm, wide black highly glossy, laterally compressed and oval or oblong in shape, they have bitter taste and strong aromatic odour.

Parts used: Seeds (detoxified form)

Chemical constituents:

The seed pulp contains 1.5% Chaksine and Isochaksine, various oils, various alkaloids and minerals like calcium, phosphorous, iron, zinc, manganese, vitamins like thiamine and riboflavin, protein, fat, sugars, tannin and mucilage.

Mizaj: Hot and dry Third/Second degree

Pharmacological actions:

Seed: Anti Inflammatory, Dessicative, Astringent, Opthalmic Tonic, Hemostyptic, Blood Purifier, Astringent, Detergent, Diuretic, Emmenogogue etc.

Unani mechanism of action:

Detergent, Diuretic, Anti Inflammatory, Dessicative properties of chaksu helps in blood purification.

Therapeutic uses:

Dysmenorrhea, Amenorrhea, Hematuria, Ring Worm, Leucoderma, Eye disorder like poor eye sight, Pterygium, Epiphora, Granular conjunctivitis, Dermatitis of eye lashes etc, chaksu is used with Zafran mamira

Dose: 2 to 3 gm

Mode of Use

For Impurities in blood it is used with sandal or kath in *keshanda* (mixing and soaking the crushed/ whole drugs overnight in water the mixture is rubbed, strained and used afterwards).

In Wound it is applied external on the form of ointment.

Infusion of chasku is useful in Leprosy

For Hematuria 21 seed of *chaksu* number with *sandal safed* 5 gm one night soaked in water, drinking in the morning relieves hematuria.

In eye diseases it is used as surma.

In bleeding piles it is used with rasaut orally. Both rasaut and chasku is powderd and tablet is made and advised one tablet twice a day.

Research Studies

Antihypertensive effect, Relaxant, Antioxidant activity, Anti-inflammatory

Antibacterial, Antifungal, Antiglycation assay, Antidiabetic activity

Anti hyperglycemic activity, α- amylase inhibitory activity.

Toxicity: Hot temperament (should be used after tadbeer)

Corrective: *Arq gulab*/corriander

Substitutes: *Totiya kirmani* (eye disorders), babchi(skin)

Compound formulations: Habbe surkhebada, habbe musaffie khon banushka kala, safuf chutki, shayaf zafra.

Chiraita

Vernaculars		
Arabic	:	Qamha, Qasab Farsee Persian
Urdu	:	Chiraita Talkh
Hindi	:	Kiryat Charayata
English	:	Chiretta, Indian Balmony, Bitter Stick
Latin	:	Swertia chirata Buch.
Syn.	:	Swertia perennis
Family	:	Gentianaceae

Introduction and History

Dioscorides described chraita with the name of Kalas while in *Makhzanul Advia,* Noor Kareemnamed as Kalamas Arumatius. Whole plant is therapeutically used in Unani Medicine since along.

Habit and Habitat:

Chirettaa is an erect annual medicinal herb which is a critically endangered grows at high altitudes in the sub-temperate regions of the Himalayas between 1200 and 2100 m altitudes from Kashmir to Bhutan) on the slopes of moist shady places.

Description in Unani:

It's a plant which grows up-to height of 1 meter; its branches are round, which are brown yellow or violet in colour. Leaves are elliptical in shape. Flowers are small and numerous. At the time of flowering, plants are collected. According to taste, it's of two types, shireen (sweet) and talkh (bitter). For medicinal purposes, mostly chiraita shireen is used. This plant is mainly found in India and Iran.

Botanical description:

S. chirayita is an annual/biennial herb 0.6–1.5 m tall. It has an erect, around 2–3 ft long stem, the middle portion is cylindrical, while the upper is quadrangular, with a prominent decurrent line at each angle. Its stem is orange brown or purplish in color with large continuous yellowish pith. Leaves are lanceolate, in opposite pairs, no stalks, acuminate, cordate at the base, sessile, five to seven nerved and 4 cm long. The root is simple, yellowish, somewhat oblique, or geniculate, tapering and short, almost 7–8 cm long and usually half an inch thick. Flowers are small, numerous, tetramerous, large leafy panicles, green-yellow, and tinged with purple and green or white hairs. The calyx is gamophyllous with four lobes, corolla-lobes four twisted and superimposed, united at the base where they have pairs of nectaries on each lobe covered with long hairs. Stamens 4, opposite the corolla lobe, at the base of the corolla. Ovary unilocular with ovules laminal placentation parietale; two stigmas. Capsules are egg-shaped, 2-valved with a transparent yellowish pericarp. Seeds are numerous, very small and dark brownish in color. Multi-colored corolla and the presence of nectaries support cross-pollination in S. chirayita.

Parts used: whole plant

Chemical constituents:

Xanthones and their derivatives, lignans, alkaloids, flavonoids, terpenoids, iridoids, secoiridoids, and other compounds such as chiratin, ophelicacid, palmitic acid, oleic acid, and stearic acid

Mizaj: hot dry second degree

Pharmacological actions:

Blood Purifier, Antipyretic, Stimulant, Gastro Tonic, Liver Tonic, Appetizer, Carminative, Antihelmenthic, Demulcent, Anti Inflammatory, Deobstruent.

Unani mechanism of action:

Owing to the bitter taste, demulcent, antiinflamattory and deobstruent properties it removes toxins from blood. recent scientific studies proved that bitternes properties of chiraita is attributed to one of the compound present in chiraita named amarogentin which is surprisingly most bitter compound isolated till date.

Therapeutic uses:

Hepatitis Liver Disorders, Fever Caused By Fasade Akhlat Salasa, Skin Diseases Viz. Pruritus, Leprosy, Hemorrhage Beneath The Skin, Acne, Boils, Leprosy, Urticaria, Ring Worm, Dermatitis.Digestive Problem Viz Anorexia, Ascites Constipation Diarrhea Helminthiasis 'Indigestion Dyspepsia Biliousness Cholera Gastritis, Bronchitis, Bronchial Asthma, Anaemia, Bodyache, Gout Inflammation, Jointpain, Uterine' Pain, Burning Sensation, Chronic Fever, Cold and Cough, Leucorrhoea, Melancholia, Morning Sickness, Oedema, Renal Colic, Scabies, Sciatica, Scorpion Stings, Poisoning, Spermatorrhoea, Wakness

Dose: 5 to 7gm

Mode of Use:

It's decoction is used in leprosy, syphilis, scabies, pruritus, abdominal cramps, indigestion, diarrhea, anorexia and seasonal fever.

Application of powderd chiraita on armpit for bad smell.

For psychological disorder its is used with karafs.

With honey it is beneficial in ascites.

Local application with rose oil and vinegar gives benfits in burns.

Research Studies:

Topo isomerase inhibition, Chemo-Preventive, Antileishmanial Effects, Anti-Inflammatory, Anesthetic, Antihistaminic, Anticonvulsant Properties, Hypotensive, Antipsychotic, Lenitive, Diuretic, Antimalarial, Antiamoebic, Antibacterial Properties, Antimalarial, Hypoglycemic, Hepatoprotective, Pro-Heamatopoitic, Chemo Preventive, Analgesic Property.

Toxicity: Kidney

Corrective: Anisoon

Substitutes: Shahatra

Compound formulations: Majun Shahtra, Arq Musaffie, Jawarish jalinus, Roghan mujarrib, Jawarish zarunni Ambary Banushkakala,

Chob Chini

Vernaculars

Arabic	:	Jazar Seenee, Fushagh Seenee
Persian	:	Chobchini
Urdu	:	Chobchini
Hindi	:	Chopchini, Chobchini, Topchini
English	:	China Root, Chinese Smilax
Latin	:	Smilax china DC.
Family	:	Liliaceae / Smilacaceae

Introduction and History

Since ancient time sarsaparilla has been used as a blood purifier and general tonic and also has been used worldwide for gout, syphilis, gonorrhea, rheumatism, wounds, venereal disease, arthritis, fever, cough, scrofula, hypertension, indigestion, psoriasis, skin diseases, and cancer. Since 1536 the *Smilax* genus is used for syphilis and other sexually-transmitted diseases throughout the world particularly in European country. With its reputation as a blood purifier, it was registered as an official herb in the U.S. Pharmacopoeia as a syphilis treatment from 1820 to 1910.

Habit and Habitat: Shrub thickets in hills and mountains. Forests, thickets, hillsides, grassy slopes, shaded places along valleys or streams from near sea level to 2000 meters.

Description in Unani: well known root cultivated in china, Japan, Nepal and Assam. Root is large, reddish pink in colour, sweet in taste and odorless. Leaves are similar to Bay Leaf. Identification of high-quality chobchini are; similar in colour externally and internally, smooth in texture, heavy in weight (should settled down in water), average in size, should not be very hard.

Botanical description: Smilax china DC is a woody vine armed with small thorns all over the stem. Rhizomes are long, thick and grey colored. Leaves are simple, alternate, elliptically oblong to subrounded, 5 to 8 centimeters long, 2.5 to 4 centimeters wide; those toward the end of the branches are much smaller and veined. Petioles are about 7 millimeters long, with adnate spiculate stipules which frequently are extended into tendrils. Inflorescence arises from the upper leaf axils, 3 to 5 centimeters long. Flowers are white to yellowish-green, their pedicels subtended by bracteoles, umbellate. Berries are globose, reddish when ripe.

Parts used: root

Chemical constituents: Phytochemical screening of methanol extract yielded flavonoids, tannins, alkaloids, saponins, and glycosides. Root contains fat, sugar, glucoside, coloring matter, gum, starch, smilacin, tannin, resin, cinchonin and saponin. Dried rhizomes yield fat, sugar, glycoside, glycoside, coloring matter, saponin, tannin, cinchonin. smilacin, and starch. Research on rhizomes yielded 13 compounds and identified kaemperol-7-O-beta-D-glucopyranoside, engeletin, isoengeletin, kaempferol, dihydrokaempferol, dihydrokaempferol-5-O-P-D-glucopyranoside, rutin, kaempferol-5-O-beta-D-glucopyranoside, 3, 5, 4'-trihydroxystibene, vanillic acid, 3, 5-dimethoxy4-O-beta-D-glu-copyranosylcinnamic acid, beta-sitosterol, and beta-daucosterol.

Mizaj: hot dry second degree

Pharmacological actions:

Root: root is Alterative, Anti-arthritic, Anti-asthmatic, Anti-bilious, Anti-flatulent, Anti-gout, Anti-paralytic, Anti-pyretic, Anti-syphilitic, Aphrodisiac, Blood Purifier, Carminative, Demulcent, Deobstruent, Desiccative, Diaphoretic, Diuretic, Emmenagogue, Hepatoprotective, Immunostimulant, Resolvent, Sedative, Stomachic and Tonic.

Unani mechanism of action:

Many times we observed that blood becomes impure and thick due to khilt sawda as chob chini owe the properties of nafe amraze sawdawiyah (beneficial in melanocholic diseases) along with mulattif (demulcent), mufattah (deobstruent), muhallil awram (resolvent), muarriq(diaphoretic) and muaddil (Alterative) properties, it purifies cleans the blood from toxic sawda.

Therapeutic uses:

Chronic diseases caused by blood (blood impurities), Leprosy, Syphilis, Wound, Ichthyosisat, Scabies, Cancrum, Pitryasis, Leucoderma, Melasma/cholasma, Pruritus, Bolis, Abscess, Ring worm, Psoriasis, Anemia with hypoprotenemia, Insomnia, Retention of urine, Dropsy, Eczema, Headache, Migraine, Bilious fever, Chronic headache, Arthritis, Lack of concentration, Renal obstructions, Chorea, Polyuria, Seminal weakness, Pruritis, Bleeding piles, Epilepsy, Rheumatism, Diarrhoea, Melancholia, Paralysis and gout, Anasarca, Malencholia, Mania, Phlebitis, Alopecia, Atrabilious jaundice.

Dose: 5 to 7 gm

Mode of Use: oral

Research Studies:

Anti-HIV -1 activity anti-HIV -1 activity, Antioxidant, Antimicrobial, Anticonvulsant, Neurotoxic effects, Anticonvulsant and neurotoxic effects, Anticonvulsant, Neurotoxic effects, Antihyperuricemic, Nephroprotective activity, Anti-inflammatory activity, Anti-nociceptive activities, Promoting blood circulation, Anti-obesity activity, Endothelial Dysfunction study, Anti-metastatic activity on Human breast cancer cells, Testicular antioxidant activity and spermatological parameters.

Toxicity: hot temprament

Corrective: Rose and Salix Caprea

Substitutes: *Smilax aristolochiaefolia*

Compound formulations: Majun chob chini, Sharbat murakkab, A chob chini, Majun ushba, Marham aatishk

Herb/Drug Interactions: Interacts with digoxin (Lanoxin) increasing the absorption of digoxin. Sarsaparilla might also decrease the elimination of lithium from the body.

GANDHAK

Vernaculars

Arabic	:	Kibreet
Hindi	:	Gandhak
English	:	Sulphur
Faarsi.	:	Kogard
Bengali	:	Gandrog
Latin	:	Rovine

Introduction and History

The term Sulfur or Sulphur derived From the Sanskrit word "Shulvari" (Shulva + Ari) meaning enemy of shulva or copper metal (Anti-copper). The Greek and Roman were familiar with the uses of sulphur oxides in fumigation and bleaching it has been used as medicament since antiquity for the purpose of scabicidal, insecticidal, fungicidal and purgative properties.

Sulphur is a non metal element occurs in the nature in the form of pure sulphur, sulphides and sulphates. It plays an imperative role for the maintains of health as skin, connective tissues, muscles, bones, teeth and hair, also control the metabolic process which is a key factor for the body. In USm sulphur is mainly used for cosmetic purposes as treatment of various skin diseases viz; Jarb, Qooba, Kharish, Taqassure Jild, Qarha Muzmina, Busoore Labnia etc. Unani Attiba describe it's uses in classical text under the caption of amraze jildia.

Description in Unani: In Unani medicine different types of Gandhak are described viz. Gandhak aamla saar, Gandhak ka phool, Danda gandhak. The first type is mostly used internally, whereas the other types are externally used. Acid can be formed from gandhak which was first made by Zakariya Raazi.

Description:

Elemental sulfur is a bright yellow, crystalline solid at room temperature. Common naturally occurring sulfur compounds include the sulfide minerals, such as pyrite (iron sulfide), cinnabar (mercury sulfide), galena (lead sulfide), sphalerite (zinc sulfide), and stibnite (antimony sulfide); and the sulfate minerals, such as gypsum (calcium sulfate), alunite (potassium aluminium sulfate), and barite (barium sulfate). It us insoluble in water but soluble in oil.

Mizaj: Haar Yabis at 3rd Degree but according to Ibn Sina, Har Yabis at 4th Degree

Pharmacological actions:

Abortificiant, Antiinflammatory, Antiseptic, Aphrodisiac, Blood purifier, Carminative, Demulcent, Desiccant Detergent, Emenogoggue, Wound healer, Rubificiant, Scabicidal.

Mechanism of action:

As per Unani physician Sulphur makes bad khilt easily removable which may be due to its Demulcent, Desiccant, Detergent and Antiseptic properties.

Therapeutic uses:

Amenorrhea, Arthritis, Asthma, Epilepsy, Gonorrhea, Jaundice, Leprosy, Melasma, Paralysis, Piles, Productive cough, Pruritus, Rhinitis, Sciatica, Sexual debility, Spasticity, Spleen diseases, Syphilis, Tuberculosis, Whoopong cough

Mudabbar (detoxifying):

One part of Gandhak Amlasar and two parts of Raughan (Ghee) are taken in a Kadeha (laddle) and kept on a low fire. When Gandhak is melted, four parts of the milk is added. This process is repeated at least three times changing the fresh Ghee and Milk each time to obtain *Gandhak Mudabbar*.

Dose: 500 mg-1gm

Toxicity: Toxic for brain and stomach as far as its toxicity is concerned, sulphur is known to be of having low toxicity and poses very little if any risk to human health. Sulfa drugs, i.e Sulfonamides can cause adverse drug reactions; the most common adverse reaction is ranging from various benign rashes to life threatening'Stevens-Johnson Syndrome'. However incidence of this 'sulfa allergy' is approximately only 3%s far as its toxicity is concerned, sulphur is known to be of having low toxicity and poses very little if any risk to human health. Sulfa drugs, i.e. Sulfonamides can cause adverse drug reactions; the most common adverse reaction is ranging from various benign rashes to life threatening 'Stevens-Johnson Syndrome'. However incidence of this 'sulfa allergy' is approximately only 3% sulfonamides can cause adverse drug reactions; the most common adverse reaction is ranging from various benign rashes to life threatening 'Stevens-Johnson Syndrome'. However incidence of this 'sulfa allergy' is approximately only 3%.

Corrective: kateera

Substitutes: one type is substitute for another.

Compound formulations:

Sayyal kibreet, marham e ushaq, dawa e siyah mushil, habbe qoobah, Zimade Jarb, Zimae Niqaras, Zimade Aateshak, Roghan gandhak, Habbe Kibreet, Marhame Kibreet, safoofe Mameeran.

Gul E Surkh

Vernaculars

Arabic	:	ward
Persian	:	Gul e surkh
Urdu	:	Gulab
Hindi	:	Gulab
English	:	Persian rose
Latin	:	Rosa damascena
Syn	:	Rosa banksia
Family	:	Rosaceae

Introduction and History

Rose is a famous and common plant. The flower of R. damascena as the king of flowers has been the symbol of love, purity, faith and beauty since the ancient times

Habit and habitat:

It is a plant of 3- 14 feet high. Leaves are dark green in colour and leaflets have usually serrated margin. Often a few small prickles on the underside of the stem. Most species have five petals and is usually white or pink, though in a few species yellow or red. Sour or sweet in taste. Most species are native to Pakistan, India, Iran, Syria with smaller numbers native to Europe, north America and north western Africa.

Botanical description:

R. damascena is a perennial bushy shrub reaching approximately 1 to 2 meters in height with large, showy and colorful flowers. The leaves are imparipinnate and compound with 5-7 leaflets Leaves are dark green colour, leaflets are serrated. Flowers are usually pink or white.

Part used: Flower, spores

Chemical constituents:

Terpenes, glycosides, flavonoids, anthocyanins, arboxylic acid, myrcene, vitamin C, kaempferol and quarcetin are found in rose. Flowers also contain a bitter principle, tanning matter, fatty oil and organic acids. itronellol, geraniol, nerol, phenyl ethyl alcohol, nonadecane, nonadecene, eicosane, heneicosane, tricosane, a-guaiene, geranyl acetate and eugenol have been reported from different parts of world.

Mizaj: Cold and dry second degree/ Murakkabul quwa

Pharmacological action:

Vital organs tonic, body tonic, stomach and intestine tonic, exhillarant, astringent, purgative, febrifuge, diaphoretic, anti inflammatory, analgesic, cicatrizant and improves complexion.

Unani mechanism of action: because of its exhilarant and Vital organs tonic property it purifies *roohe haiwani* and *roohe nafsani* ultimately resulting in strengthening of heart and brain. It removes toxins from the skin pore because of its Diaphoretic activity. stomach and intestine tonic leads to improvement in the performance of stomach and intestine.

Therapeutic uses:

External use: used in conjunctivitis, used in ear aches, headache, prevent toothache, used in oral ulcers, prevent excessive perspiration, used in stomatitis.

Internal use:

Palpitation and syncope, prevent weakness of heart, strengths stomach, intestine, liver, used in epistaxis, hepatomegaly, pericarditis, hepatitis, constipation, headache.

Dose : 5- 7 gm

Mode of use:

Rose is used as safoof in inflammation of visceras such as hepatitis, gastritis, inflammation of uterus and endocarditis and weakness of stomach and intestine.

Inhalation of fresh flower is worked as an exhillarant and tonic to heart and brain but in debilitated person it stimulate coryza.

Pressed out water of rose is used in conjunctivitis by qutoor and also used in ear ache.

It's zimad is used in awaram e harra such as hepatitis and headache.

Safoof is externally applied on body to prevent perspiration and provides fragrance.

Massage of roghan e gulis used in dissolution of swelling.

Joshanda of root is used in joint pain, syphilis and wound.

Safoof of flower is used in piles and also used in aphrodisiac.

Safoof of seeds is used in menorrhagia and leucorrhoea.

Its leaves used in ascitis and jaundice.

Research Studies

Antimicrobial effects, Analgesic effect, Anticancer activity, Anticonvulsant, Anti-depressant, Anti-diabetic, Anti-HIV, Anti-inflammatory effect, Antioxidant activity, Antitussive effect, Anxiety, Bronchodilatory, Depressant activity, Hr and contractility, Hypnotic, Laxative and prokinetic, Protective effects on neuritic atrophy, Relaxant.

Toxicity: cough and thirst

Corrective: Anisun

Substitutes: Banafsha

Compound formulations:

Shabrbar ward, Gulqand, Majun Dabeedul ward, Dawaul misk, Roghan gul, Sharbat Ahmad Shahi, Safi, Mufarrah sheikh ur raees, Jawarish zarishk.

Halela Siyah

Vernaculars		
Arabic	:	Halilaj aswad
Persian	:	Halela zangi
Hindi	:	Kaali harr
English	:	Black myrobalan
Latin	:	Terminalia chebula
Syn.	:	Buceras chebula (Retz.) Lyons Combretum argyrophyllum K.Schum. Myrobalanus chebula (Retz.) Gaertn.
Family	:	Combretaceae

Introduction and History

Terminalia chebula Retz. (Fam. Combretaceae), is called the 'King of Medicine' in Tibet and is always listed at the top of the list of 'Ayurvedic Materia Medica'. The whole plant possesses high medicinal value and traditionally used for the treatment of various ailments for human beings. Some of the folklore people used this plant in the treatment of asthma, sore throat, vomiting, hiccough, diarrhea, dysentery, bleeding piles, ulcers, gout, heart and bladder diseases. The plant has been demonstrated to possess multiple pharmacological and medicinal activities.

Habit and Habitat:

Terminalia chebula is found throughout South East Asia including in India, Sri Lanka, Bhutan, Nepal, Bangladesh, Myanmar, Cambodia, Laos, Vietnam, Indonesia, Malaysia, Pakistan and Thailand. In China, it is native in W Yunnan and cultivated in Fujian, Guangdong, Guangxi (Nanning), and Taiwan (Nantou).

In India, it is found in the Sub Himalayan region from Ravi eastwards to West Bengal and Assam, ascending up to the altitude of 1,500 m (4,900 ft) in the Himalayas. This tree is wild in forests of Northern India, central provinces and Bengal, common in Madras, Mysore and in the southern part of the Bombay presidency. Its habitat includes dry slopes up to 900 m (3,000 ft) in elevation.

Botanical description:

Terminalia chebula is a medium to large deciduous tree growing to 30 m (98 ft) tall, with a trunk up to 1 m (3 ft 3 in) in diameter. The leaves are alternate to subopposite in arrangement, oval, 7–8 cm (2.8–3.1 in) long and 4.5–10 cm (1.8–3.9 in) broad with a 1–3 cm (0.39–1.18 in) petiole. They have an acute tip, cordate at the base, margins entire, glabrous above with a yellowish pubescence below. The fruit is drupe-like, 2–4.5 cm (0.79–1.77 in) long and 1.2–2.5 cm (0.47–0.98 in) broad, blackish, with five longitudinal ridges. The dull white to yellow flowers are monoecious, and have a strong, unpleasant odour. They are borne in terminal spikes or short panicles. The fruits are smooth ellipsoid to ovoid drupes, yellow to orange-brown in colour, with a single angled stone.

Unani description:

Terminalia chebula Retz (Halela siyah) is a medium to large deciduous tree found all over India, mostly in areas of light rainfall. It grows upto 25-30m in height. Flowers are white or yellow in colour with a strong unpleasant odour, borne in a terminal spikes. Leaves are small, elliptic rhombus, with an acute tip, glabrous above and yellowish pubescence below. The author of the Makhzan-ul-Advia has stated that it has six varieties, the very young fruit is about the size of cumin seeds are called Halileh-i- zira; when its size becomes a grain of barley, Halileh-i-jawi; when the size of a raisin, Halileh-i-zangi or hindi; when yellowish and half arrived at maturity, Halileh-i-chini; when further developed, Halileh-i-asfar; and lastly when relatively mature, Halileh-i-kabuli. The second, third and last variety of chebulic myrobalans are used for medicinal purposes.

Mizaj: Cold 1 Dry 2

Part used: Fruit

Chemical constituents:

Myrobaline, Tannin, Chebulic acid, Tannic acid, Gallic acid, Resin, methyl gallate, ethyl gallate, chebulagic acid, tetra-O-galloyl-β-D-glucose, and ellagic acid, chebulinic acid and penta-O galloyl-β-D-glucose. Ellagitannin such as punacalagin, casurarinin, corilagin and terchebulin and others such as chebulanin, neochebulinic acid, chebulagic acid and chebulinic acid have been reported to be associated with the plant. The triterpenes have been reported which are arjun glucoside 1, arjungenin and the chebulosides 1 and 2.

Pharmacological actions:

Melanagogue (mushile sauda), brain tonic (muqawwie dimagh), Muqawwie basar (eye tonic), blood purifier, stomach tonic, Astringent, Hair blackener, Muqaawi meda, muqawwi ama, jazib.

Unani mechanism of action:

Sawda being the commonest cause of blood impurities and haleela is the drug of choice for removing impure sawda, it cleans the blood from toxic sawda.

Therapeutic use:

Leprosy, palpitation, anxiety, splenomegaly, indigestion, arthritis, fever, melancholia, ascities, piles, bleeding and loose gums and also gums ulceration, wounds and ulcers. Conjunctivitis, oral ulcers, sore throat and stomatitis, bleeding gums, hair wash and cleaning tooth in pyorrhea. Several gastrointestinal ailments such as ascites, tumors, enlargement of liver-spleen, piles, colitis and intestinal, digestion and improves appetite.

Mode of use:

Its powder is used in weak memory, saudawi amraz, melancolea, piles, leprosy, stomach and intestinal weakness, loose motions.

Its decoction or joshanda is used in weakened eyesight, brain disorders, safrawi diseases.

It is also used in the form of murabba.

Research studies:

Antioxidant and free radical scavenging activity, Anticarcinogenic activity, Antimutagenic, radioprotective and chemopreventive activity, Hepatoprotective activity, Cardioprotective activity, Cytoprotective activity, Antidiabetic and renoprotective activity, Antibacterial activity, Antifungal activity, Antiviral activity, Antiprotozoal activity, Anti-inflammatory and anti-arthritic activity, Adaptogenic and antianaphylactic activities, Hypolipidemic and hypocholesterolemic acivity, Gastrointestinal motility improving and anti-ulcerogenic activity, Antispasmodic activity, Anticaries activity, Wound healing activity, Purgative property, Immunomodulatory activity, Anti-allergic activity.

Dosage:

Joshanda (decoction) in the dose of 30 ml to 80 ml.

Powder. 3 -7 gms

Toxicity: tenesmus

Correctives: Honey, jujube (unnab), Almond oil

Substitute: Halela zard, Halela kaabuli

Compound formulations:

Itrifalaat, Safoof Muqliyasa, Safoof chutki, Majoon muqul.

Hiran Khuri

Vernaculars

Arabic	:	Lablab -al- haqaul
Persian	:	Pechak sehrayi
Urdu	:	Lehli, Wanvehri, Baily
Hindi	:	Hiran khuri
English	:	Field bindweed
Latin	:	Convolvulus arvensis
Syn.	:	Convolvulus chinensis Ker Gawl
Family	:	Convolvulaceae

Introduction and History

Hiran khuri is used since ancient times for the treatment of various ailments.

Habit and Habitat:

Bindweed is a prostrate or climbing perennial herb. It has weak stem but powerful root system that may cover an area 6m diameter and extend to a depth of 9m.It is generally distributed over Africa and south America, south east Asia and pacific islands. Although the plant can be found in waste areas, it can also grow in all kinds of cultivated lands. It grows best on rich, fertile soils but persists on poor and gravely soils as well.

Description in Unani:

It is a small twining perennial herb. It has very thin branches as threads. It's leaves are like a mark of deer's foot but smaller and longer than that Flowers are bowl-like but pinkish white in colour. The herb is spicy in taste. It's flower has no fragrance, while chewing it's leaf or flower they act as a minor irritant to mouth, and then in lubricates the mouth.

Botanical description:

It is a creeping herb. It's roots are very deep taproot 0.5-3 m or more long. It's stem is slender, smooth to hairy, 1 to 3 m long, twining or spreading over the soil surface. The rhizomes are cordlike and fleshy, which permeate the soil in all directions. It's shoot buds reach the surface and establish new crowns. Leaves are ulternate, simple, long-petiolated, margins entire, ovate-oblong, narrowing gradually upward to the rounded or blunt tip, the base squarish or the lobes pointing downward or concavely toward the stalk, smooth to slightly hairy, up to 6cm long & 3cm wide.

Flowers usually borne singly in the axils of the leaves, flower stalk one to four flowered, slender, up to 6cm or longer, with two bracts 1cm to 2.5 cm below the flower. Sepals bell shaped, 3mm long. Fruit is capsule ovate, two or four seeded. Seeds are three-angled, ovoid, dull, dark brownish grey to black, 3mm to 5mm long.

Parts used: Whole herb is used.

Chemical constituents:

It contains alkaloids, phenolic compounds, sterols, resin. It is a good source of flavanoids, carbohydrates, sugars, mucilage. It also has tannins, unsaturated sterols/triterpenes, lactones and protiens. onvolvulus arvensis was found to contain the tropane alkaloids, tropine, pseudotropine, tropinone as well as cuscohygrine, meso-cuscohygrine and calystegines. vannilic, syringic, benzoic and salicylic acids were detected in the phenolic acids fraction. Many researchers mentioned that the plant contained four coumarins, 7-hydroxycoumarin (umbelliferone); 6,7- dihydroxycoumarin (esculetin); 6-methoxy-7-hydroxycoumarin (scopoletin) and 6-methoxycoumarin7-O- glucoside (scopoletin7-O-glucoside), and eleven flavonoids including Kaempferol and its 3-O-β-D-glucoside, 7- O-β-D-glucoside, 3-O-α-L-rhamnosyl, 7-O-β-D-glucoside, 3-O-rutinoside, 7-O-rutinoside, 3-O-α-L-rhamnoside and 3-O-β-D-galactorhamnoside as well as Quercetin and its 3-O-α-L-rhamnoside and 3-O-rutinoside.

Mizaj: Hot, Dry (some says Hot, Wet also)

Pharmacological actions:

Blood purifier, hepato-protective, anti-diarrheal, diuretic, antidote, anti-inflammatory, concoctive.

Unani mechanism of action:

It maintains the temperament of blood due to its "musaffi-e-damm" property. It maintains homeostasis of the body due to it's diuretic (mudirr-e- bol) property. It maintains the blood pressure by vasodialating effect. It prevents the poisonous effect of mouse-biting due to it's antidote (faad-e-zeher) property, it works when it is dried and inhaled through nose, so that the poisonous air will escape or will be cleansed. It's "joshanda" eleminates "safra, balgham & sawda" due to it's hepato-protective (Muqavvi-e-jigar) property.

Therapeutic Uses:

It dries excessive fluid in the brain and hence cures "amraz-e-ratab" of brain.

It is used in eye diseases, coryza and coug, blood disease eg. Haemorrhage, leprosy, itching and acne, diabetes, hepatitis, acidity and piles, reduced sperm count and low viscosity.

Dose: 7gm to 12gm.

Mode of use:

Hiran khuri 2.5 gm with coriander leaves's water is beneficial in dysentery.

Misri and hiran khuri in equal quantity relives all kind of blood diseases.

3 gm of hiran khuri when taken orally relieves itching.

By dropping it inside nasal cavity, it dries excess fluid in the brain.

By making it's water or "jal" and applying on eyes, it strengthens the eyesight.

It's "joshanda" prevents from Cough & Coryza.

After a good mixing when it is taken as a liquid it prevents piles.

It prevents Hepatitis when it's juice is dropped into eyes.

It's powder or "sufoof" orally prevents diabetes.

It's powder when taken orally is potent for reproductive system.

It is dried and taken as steam so that bad and poisonous air is pured.

Research Studies:

A lot of research studies have been carried out on this drug:

Anti-bacterial, Immuno-stimulant, Anti-diarrheal, Anti-diabetic, Antioxidant effect, Vasodilating effect, Immunostimulant effect, Hepato-protective, Anti-angiogenesis, Cytotoxic.

Toxicity:

It is a strong lexative in high amounts. Large amounts can cause stomach pain.

Corrective: Honey

Substitute: Not known

Compound Formulations:

Joshanda hiran khuri, Hubb-e-hiran khuri, Kajal hiran khuri, Ghota hiran khuri, Namak hiran khuri.

MUNDI

Vernaculars

Arabic	:	Kamazriyus
Persian	:	Kamaduriyus
Urdu	:	Gule Mundi
Hindi	:	Gorakh Mundi, Mundi
English	:	East Indian Globe-thistle
Latin	:	Sphaeranthus indicus Linn
Syn.	:	*S. senegalensis* DC./ *S. hirtus*Willd
Family	:	Asteraceae

Introduction and History

Mundi is a well known medicinal plant widely used in Unani system of medicine for curing various ailments.

Habit and Habitat: It is found abundantly in damp situations in the plains all over India, ascending to an altitude of 1500 m in the hills, especially as a weed in the rice-fields.

Description in Unani:

It is an Indian origin Grass. Leaves looks like mint. Stem is spread on earth. It is of two types small and large. Small also known as ghundi flower is of red colour and looks similar to rose. Second variety is big flower looks like wheat flower. Also known as maha mundi. Small variety is more effective.

Botanical description

A spreading aromatic herb, about 30-60 cm tall with glandular, hairy, winged stems, wings toothed. Leaves sessile, decurrent, obovate-oblong, spinous serrate, narrow at the base. Flowers purple, in close terminal, globose or ovoid heads.Achenes glabrous, stalked.

Parts used: Whole plant

Chemical constituents: bitter alkaloid, sphaeranthine, has been reported in the plant. Capitula contains albumin, a fatty oil (up to 5%), reducing sugars, tannins, mineral matter, a volatile oil (0.007%), and a glucoside. The flower contains sesquiterpene glycoside, sphaeranthanolide, beta-D-glucoside of beta-sitosterol, aglycone, stigmasterol, *n*-triacontanol, *n*-pentacosane and hentriacontane. Eudesmanolides, cryptomeridiol and 4-epicryptomeridiol have been isolated from flowers.

Mizaj: hot wet second degree

Pharmacological actions: Astringent, tonic to vital organ, tonic to stomach, appetizer, blood purifier, demulcent, tonic to eye, anti catarrh, anti inflammatory, anti tumor, protective for eye sight, nervine tonic, cardiac tonic, antihelmintic.

Unani mechanism of action:

It is observed that blood becomes impure and thick due to khilt sawda as Mundi owe the properties of nafe amraze sawdawiyah (beneficial in melanocholic diseases) along with mulattif (demulcent), tonic to stomach, muhallil awram (resolvent), **properties,** it purifies cleans the blood from toxic sawda.

Therapeutic uses:

Cardiac debility, Melancholia, Epiphora, Cholera, Dyssentries, Hypertrophy of prostarte gland, Palpitation, Premature graying of hair, Safrawi and saudawi diseases, Indigestion, Inflammation, Pruritus, Ringworm, Leprosy, Boils, Abscess, Gonorrehea, Gout, Sciatica, Intestinal worms, Bleeding piles, Cough, Nervine weakness.

Dose: 1 to 7 gm

Mode of Use:

In cutaneous diseases like boils, abscess, ring worm etc mundi can be used in powder form, decoction form orally.

When taken orally with haleela and amla it rejuvenates body.

Eating Halwa made by mundi for 40 consecutive days blackens hair and stops hair fall.

Research Studies:

Anthelmintic activity, Antibacterial, Anticancer activity, Antiprotozoal activity against *Entamoeba histolytica,* Antidiabetic activity, Antifeedant activity, Antifungal, Antihyperlipidemic activity, Anti-inflammatory activity, Antimicrobial activity, Antioxidant activity, Antipyretic activity, Antitussive activity, Antiviral activity, Anxiolytic activity, Attenuation effect on prostatic hypertrophy, Bronchodilatory Effect, Deterrant activity, Hepatoprotective activity, Immunomodulatory activity, Larvicidal action, Macrofilaricidal activity, Mast cell Stabilizing effect, Mosquito repellent, Nephroprotective effect, Neuroleptic activity, Ovicidal activity, Psychotropic activity, Repellent, Wound healing activity.

Toxicity: hot temprament

Corrective: Bhangra

Substitutes: Sarphuka

Compound formulations: Naqu shahtra, Arq musafiie khun, Itrifal mundi, Majun mundi, Tiryaq faruq, Arq mundi.

Neel Kanthi

Vernaculars

Urdu	:	Neel kanthi
Hindi	:	karu
English	:	Indian gentian
Latin	:	Gentianodes kurroo
Syn.	:	Gentiana kurroo Royle
Family	:	Gentianaceae

Introduction and History

The name Gentiana is derived from "Gentius" a king of Illyria (Europe), who is believed to have discovered the medicinal value of the Gentian root. In fact, the specific name of G. kurroo Royle is from the local name for the root of the plant, "Karu" meaning bitter.

Habit and Habitat:

A perennial rhizomatous herb, up to 25cm tall, found in temperate and sub-alpine zones. The species is distributed in the Himalayan region across India, Pakistan and Nepal. It is endemic to the north-western Himalayas and commonly grows in Kashmir, Himachal Pradesh, and adjoining hills of the north-western Himalayas.

Description in Unani:

It is a plant found mostly in hilly regions. It don't have branches and stem. Leaves are oval and green from one side and red and rough from another side. Flowers are blue in colour. Taste is bitter.

Botanical description:

Stem glabrous branched from base. Leaves simple, basal leaves oblong-linear, entire, acute, univeined. Cauline leaves linear, entire and acute.Inflorescence terminal, 1-3 flowered. Flower showy, dark blue, bell shaped. Calyx lobes linear, entire, acute. Corolla blue speckled with white. Lobes ovate, entire and acute. Fruit a capsule, stalked. Seed numerous, oval. small perennial herb with tufted decumbent stems, 10 – 13 cm high. Rootstock stout and thick. Leaves radical rosulate, narrowly oblong lanceolat or elliptic-lanceolate, spathulate, subacuteacute, coriaceous, purplish on dorsal surface, 3 – 13.5 x 0.3 – 1.5 cm; nerves 1 – 3, midrib prominent on dorsal side, base connate into 5 – 9 mm long tubes; margins revolute, crenulate. Flowers blue with white spots, terminal, solitary-subsolitary, often 3-clustered, pedicellate, 5-merous, 2.4 – 5.5 x 1 – 3.2 cm, pedicels 5-lineolate, 0.8 – 3 cm long. Seeds numerous.

Parts used: whole plant

Chemical constituents:

iridoids, xanthones, C-glucoxanthone mangiferin, and C-glucoflavones

Mizaj: Hot wet and according to some Hot dry 2

Pharmacological actions:

Anti-infammatory, analgesic, anticonvulsant, hypotensive, antipsychotic, sedative, diuretic, antimalarial, anti-amoebic and antibacterial.

Unani mechanism of action:

Taste is bitter and temperament is hot and has a number of pharmacological properties viz. anti-infammatory etc. By virtue of these characteristics it is able to convert the morbid viscous matter into such a form which can be easily evacuated by the body and diuretic properties help in removing from the body.

Therapeutic uses:

Cough, fever, headache, liver ailments and as a blood purifier. The drug obtained from G. kurroo is very helpful in removing all kinds of weakness and overtiredness of body from prolonged illness, recovers digestive system and lack of appetite. In the Unani system of medicine, the flower tops (Gule-Ghafis) are used for treatment of inflammation, pain, antipyretic and hepatitis and in the preparation of tonics for stomachic. It is also curative for the skin disease leucoderma, leprosy, dyspepsia, colic, anorexia, flatulence, helminthiosis, anti-inflammatory, amenorrhea, dysmenorrhoeal, haemorrhoids, strangury, constipation, urinary infections as an antiseptic, bitter tonic, cholagogue and bronchial asthma.

Dose: 5-7 grms

Mode of Use:

leaf powder of G. kurroo (Neilkanth) is mixed with oil and is applied on ulcer and fungal infection. However, the root of G. kurroo is used in stomach-ache and in urinary infections; the root with ginger root powder is also used for curing high fevers.

Research Studies:

Research studies shows it has anti bacterial, anti oxidant, anti arthriic and anti inflammatory, analgesics, anti diebetic activity.

Toxicity:

Corrective: Honey

Substitutes: Barham dandi

Compound formulations:

NEEM

Vernaculars		
Arabic	:	Neeb
Persian	:	Azad Darakhte
Urdu	:	Neem
Hindi	:	Neem, Nimb
English	:	Indian Lilac, Neem, Margosa
Latin	:	Azadirachta indica A. Juss./
Syn.	:	*Melia azadirachta* Linn.
Family	:	Meliaceae

Introduction and History

Neem is well known and used for its medicinal properties from ancient period (4000 BC); being very popular, even revered worldwide. Neem also known as legendary medicinal tree of India. Latinized name of Neem Azadirachta indica is derived from the Persian word Azad meaning Free and dirakht meaning Tree, i stands for Hind (Indian Origin) which literally means the free tree of India.

Habit and Habitat:

Neem, is a large, evergreen tree, 12-18m in height and 1.8-2.4m in girth, with a straight and long, spreading branches forming a board crown, commonly found throughout the greater part of India.

Description in Unani:

Neem is a large found wild and often cultivated in India. The height of the tree is about 12 meters to 15 meters. All the part of the tree is bitter in taste. Its stem is erect and having a girth of 1.75 meters to 2.75 meters with spreading branches. Bark is dark grey and rough Leaves are green in color, bluntly serrate and alternate. The flowers are white, having a scented odor especially at night. Its fruit is smooth, oblong and small in size and is called, Nicola. Unripe fruit is color and bitter in taste while the ripe fruit is yellow colored and somewhat sweetish in taste. Its four varieties viz. Ban, Bakain (Maha neem), Bhoin neem and Meetha neem (Kiryapak) have been mentioned in classical literature.

Botanical description:

The leaves are alternate, impair pinnate and 20-38 cm long. The leaflets are 8-19 cm alternate or opposite. Leaves are ovate-lanceolate, oblique or sub foliate, glossy and bluntly serrate. The flowers are hermaphrodite, white or pale yellow, small, scented and numerous. Flowers are very lax and in axillary panicles. The calyx is five lobed. The sepals are small in size. The petals are five in number, polypetalous. Stamina tube is a little shorter than the petals. There are 9-10 lobes at the apex; the lobes are truncate, again slightly toothed. The anthers are within the tube opposite to and shorter than the lobes.

Parts used: leaves, fruit, bark of stem and root, kernel, sap

Chemical constituents:

Neem is rich in margosic acid, nimbin, nimbidin, nimbinene. azadirachtin, meliantrol, salanin, quercetin (flavonoid) and nimbosterol (ß- sitosterol) as well as number of liminoids (nimbin and its derivatives). Neem contains protein (7.1%), carbohydrates (22.9%), minerals, calcium, phosphorus, vitamin C, carotene etc. But they also contain glutamic acid, tyrosine, aspartic acid, alanine, praline, glutamine and cystine like amino acids, and several fatty acids (dodecanoic, tetradecanoic, elcosanic, etc.).

Mizaj: hot and dry first degree/ cold first degree dry second degree

Pharmacological actions:

Various Pharmacological action described in Unani Classical literature are as follows,

Resolvent, Analgesic, Laxative, Concoctive, Anti Pyretic, Anti Septic, Anti Helmenthic, Blood Tonic, Anti Inflammatory, Clears Safra, *Balgham* and flatulence, Digestive, Stimulant To Blood Circulation, Antiseptic, Antipyretic, Emmanagogue, Cicatrizant,

Thirst quenching, Eye tonic, Antitussive, Antidiarrheal, Anti hydrotic, Anti Diabetic Repellent Anti rheumatic

Unani mechanism of action:

Since its taste of neem is very bitter and temperament is hot in addition it has a number of pharmacological properties viz. demulcent, laxative, resolvent, deobstruent, diuretic, antiseptic etc. By virtue of these characteristics it is able to transform the morbid viscous matter into such a form which can be easily evacuated by the body.

Therapeutic uses:

Abscess, Chronic arthritis, Dandruff, diabetes, Ear ache, Join pain, Leprosy, Leucoderma, Melasma/Cholasma, Piles, Pitryasis, Pruritus, Pustule, Ring worm, Safrawi Fever, Thread worm.Neem stick is used to remove bad smell form mouth

Dose: leaves: 7 to 10 gm

Fruit: 1 to 3 gm

Mode of Use:

Orally can be used in all skin disorder

Decoction of neem leaves poured locally on wounds which destroys smell of wound ad helps in healing.

Applying leaves on wound and ulcer heals it.

Fruit of neem clears constipation.

Pills of neem fruit are very effective in piles.

Washing hair with the water of neem fruit clears lice.

Application of neem oil is beneficial in fungal infection of skin and other skin diseases, joint pains.

Research Studies:

Acaricidal activity, Anthelmintic activity, Antibacterial activity, Anti-bovine activity, Anti-cancer effects, Anti-diabetic, Anti-hypertensive activity, Anti-inflammatory, Antimalarial activity, Anti-neoplastic activity, Anti-oxidant activity, Anti-trypanosomal, Anti-tumor activity, Antiviral, Chemotactic activity, Free radical scavenging activity, Hepatotoxicity, Immunological function, Immunostimulatory agent, Insecticidal, Larvae of *boophilus decolotatus*, Larvae of filarial, Larvicidal activity, Leukocyte adopsis, Melanogenesis inhibitory, Nutritional activity, Propylactic activity, Transmission blocking activity, Tumor cell killing.

Toxicity: Dry temperament

Corrective: Honey

Substitutes: Leaves is a substitute of fruit vice versa

Compound formulations: Majun Bawaseer, Habbe Musaffie Khoon, Arq Murakkab Musaffie Khun Ba Nushka Kala, Marham Jadwar, Safi.

Panwad

Vernaculars		
Sanskrit	:	Chakar mard
Arabic	:	Qalb
Persian	:	Sang saboya
Hindi	:	Chagond
English	:	Sickle senna
Latin	:	Cassia tora
Syn	:	Senna tora
Family	:	Fabaceae

Introduction and History

Senna tora (originally described by Linnaeus as Cassia tora) is a dicot legume in the subfamily Caesalpinioideae. Its name is derived from its Sinhala name Tor.

Habit and Habitat:

Cassia tora is found in many parts of the world. It grows abundantly in parts of Afghanistan, India, Nigeria, China, Pakistan, Myanmar, Nepal and Bhutan. It is also grown and cultivated areas in the Himalayas at the elevation of 1400 meters in Nepal. It is distributed throughout India, Sri Lanka, West China and the tropics, particularly in forest and tribal areas.

Botanical description:

The Cassia tora is an herbaceous annual foetid herb. The plant can grow 30–90 centimeters (12–35 in) tall and consists of alternative pinnate leaves with leaflets mostly with three opposite pairs that are obovate in shape with a rounded tip. The leaves grow up to 3–4.5 centimeters long. The stems have distinct smelling foliage when young. The flowers occur in pairs in axils of leaves with five petals and pale yellow in colour. The stamens are of unequal length.

The pods are somewhat flattened or four angled, 10–15 cm long and sickle shaped, hence the common name sickle pod. There are 30–50 seeds within a pod.

Unani description:

Its plant is about half guz long (12-35in). Its leaf is conical and somewhat oval in shape. Flowers are yellow in colour. Its seeds are very hard and covered in a pod.

Mizaj: Hot Dry 2

Part used: Seeds. Shoots, leaves, root.

Chemical constituents:

Fistucacidin, emodin, rubro fusarin, torosachrysone, isotoralactone, questin, obtusin, obtusifolin, alaternins, cassiaside, chrysophenol etc.

Seeds: cinnamaldehyde, gum, tannins, mannitol, coumarins, aldehydes, eugenol and pinene, sugars, resins.

Root: Beta sitosterol, Beta-D glucoside, palmitic acid, stearic acid, uridine, quercitin, iso-quercitin.

Pharmacological actions: purgative, phlegmagogue and melanagogue, blood purifier, detergent, antiepidemic, antihelmintic, anti-inflammatory, digestive, dessicative etc.

Therapeutic use:

Skin diseases like leprosy, pruritis, leucoderma, pityriasis, lentigo, ringworm, urticaria, allergic skin rashes etc. In other diseases like cough, chronic respiratory disorders, asthma, paralysis, arthritis, tumors of the abdomen, piles, worm infestation, toxicity, snake bite poisoning,

Mechanism of action: Panwad has very good detergent dessicative and digestive properties because of which it is used to purifies skin externally.

Mode of use:

Its seeds are soaked in curd for few days and its liniment is applied on ring worm.

Cooked leaves are eaten as preventive measure in endemics of plague.

Its paste with wine or vinegar locally applied in vitiligo, and other skin diseases.

Its liniment is used in ring worm.

Cooked leaves are consumed orally in epidemics of plague as preventive measure.

Orally panwar seed is used for vitiligo, pruritus, leprosy, ring worm, pityriasis etc.

Panwar seed orally and localy effective in piles.

Decoction of leaves is used in teething fever.

According to Hakeem Ali when panwar seed is dried under sun and powdered and mixed with curd if applied locally on alopecia gives good result in alopecia areata.

Research studies:

Anthelmintic activity, Antibacterial activity, Antifertility activity, Antifungal activity, Antigenotoxic properties, Anti-inflammatory effect, Antimutagenic activity, Antioxidant activity, Antiproliferative activity, Hepatoprotective activity Purgative activity, Hypolipidemic activity, Immunostimulatory activitiy, Nitric oxide scavenging activity, Oxytocic activity, Spasmogenic and Antinociceptive activity.

Dosage:

Seeds powder 4-6 g.

Toxicity: toxic to intestines

Correctives: Milk, Curd, Rose

Substitute: Babchi (psoralea seeds), beekh sarkanda

Compound formulations: Nazd qooba, zimad bars, safuf bars, majun bhangra, kaya kalp.

Sandal Surkh

Vernaculars

Arabic	:	Sandal Ahmer
Persian	:	Sandal surkh
Hindi	:	Laal chandan
English	:	Red Sandal wood
Latin	:	Pterocarpus santalinus
Syn.	:	Santalum rubrum
Family	:	Leguminosae

Introduction and History

Red sandal wood is one of most valuable trees, which have limited distribution in India. The scientific name is Latinized Ancient Greek and means “wing fruit”, referring to the unusual shape of the seed pods in this genus.

Habit and Habitat:

Its is a moderate-sized deciduous tree with clear trunk and dense rounded crown. Pterocarpus santalinus is endemic to the southern Eastern Ghats mountain range of South India.

Botanical description:

Sandal surkh is a light-demanding moderate-sized tree, growing to 8 meters (26 ft) tall with a trunk 50–150 cm diameter. It is fast-growing when young, reaching 5 meters (16 ft) tall in three years, even on degraded soils. It is not frost tolerant, being killed by temperatures of −1 °C. The leaves are alternate, 3–9 cm long, trifoliate with three leaflets. The flowers are produced in short racemes. The fruit is a pod 6–9 cm long containing one or two seeds.

Unani description:

Tree is about 10-11meters long. Its bark is blackish brown which when cut oozes out a liquid (rutubat) of red colour. Its wood is dark red in colour and has pleasant smell; this wood is used as medicine in unani medicine. Leaves are small and flowers are yellow in colour.

Mizaj: Cold second degree Dry third degree

Part used: heartwood

Chemical constituents: Pterocarpus species are found to be rich in isoflavonoids, terpenoids, and related phenolic compounds, β-sitosterol, lupeol, (-) epicatechin. glycosides viz., 6-OH-1-methyl-3',4',5'-trimethoxyaurone-4-O-rhamnoside and 6,4'-dihyroxyaurone-4-O-neohesperidoside, and isoflavone glycoside 4',5-dihydroxy 7-methyl isoflavone 3'-O-beta-*D*-glucoside are also present in P. santalinus. Santaline, glucoside, colouring matter etc. pterocarpol, santalins A and B, pterocarptriol, ispterocarpolone, pterocarpodiolones with β-eudeslol and cryptomeridol in heartwood. Ether, alkalis, and three other crystalline principles santal, pterocarpin, homopterocarpin, small quantity of tannin, and kino-tannic acid have also been found in the wood.

Pharmacological actions:

Astringent, blood purifier, Analgesic, Heart tonic, anti pyretic, refrigent, resolvent of inflammation of warm origin, sedative, diaphoretic, hepatoprotective.

Mechanism of action: many physician doubts on the blood purification properties of sandal. They claims that sandal is very much effective in sawdawi diseases due to its musakkin hiddat properties. Because of which it is listed as blood purifier.

Therapeutic use:

Dysentery, enteritis, gastririts, hepatitis, blood diarrohea, jaundicie, cystitis, high grade fever, urethririts, hematuria, burning micturation, menorrhegia, gonorrhea, diabetes, palpitation, Burning feeling and Inflammations, Poison, Bleeding.

Mode of use:

Externally: Almost all pharmacological actions are similar with sandal safaid, Externally it is more effective than sandal safaid.

Powder, paste or infusion is applied to all types of inflammation, Headache, Skin irritations, excessive sweating, Fever and Boils.

Topically it is used to strengthen the Sight and reduce selling of the eyes including conjunctivitis.

Bathing with sandal surkh detoxify blood, cleans skin.

Orally is given to treat toxins in blood, poisonos condition, burning micturation, hematuria, nausea, vomiting, etc

Paste with milk is applied on Bleeding Piles.

As a paste for skin spots, freckles and discolorations, with Madder, Costus, Symplocos racemosa and roasted Lentils,

To clears Liver Heat red sandalwood is used with White Sandalwood, Rose, Red Coral, Tabasheer and Camphor orally.

Dosage: In Powder: 2–5 grams; In Decoction: 3–9 grams

Research studies:

Analgesic, Angiogenesis and wound-healing activity, Anti cancerous activity, Anti inflammatory activity, Antifungal, antimutagenic, Antioxidant activity, Antiviral, Antiallodynic, Anti-Helicobacter pylori, Anti-hepatotoxic effects, Anti-hyperglycemic, Anti-hyperlipidemic, Anti-inflammatory, Antimicrobial activity, Antiplasmodial activity, Antipyretic activity, Gastroprotective effect, Hepatoprotective activity, Radical-scavenging.

Toxicity: decrease sexual activity

Correctives: Honey

Substitute: Sandal Safed

Compound formulations: Habbe soozak, Arq soozak, Maajoon e ushba, naqu shahtra, habbe bawasir badi, habbe musaffie khun, sharbat anjabar, majun ushba, sharbat musaffie khun.

SAMMULFAR

Vernaculars

Arabic	:	Sammul Far
Persian	:	Marg mosh
Urdu	:	Sankhia
Hindi	:	Sankhia
Latin	:	Arsenium
English	:	Arsenic
Syn.	:	White arsenic, Arsenous oxide

Introduction and History

Arsenic is a naturally occurring element. It occurs in many minerals, usually in combination with sulfur and metals. It is widely distributed in Earth's crust. It is found in water, air, food and soil. Pure arsenic is grey coloured and bright. It is brittle in nature. It is not used in medicine in pure form.

Description In Unani:

Arsenic is found in white crystal form. Arsenic is usually present in a mixed form along with iron and sulfur. It is metallic substance it's a fume of silver obtained from mine of silver, according to some obtained from gold mine and according to some it is a compound of mercury and sulphur. I Makhzanul Advia it is mentioned that according to Ved Arsenis is of five types

Mizaj: Hot and Dry 4th degree

Pharmacological Actions:

Body tonic, Nerve tonic, Stomach tonic, Antiphlegmatic, Blood purifier, Aphrodisiacs, Antipyretic, Antiseptic, Siccative, Corrosive.

Therapeutic Uses:

Used in body weakness.

Used in Ischemia.

Used in paralysis.

Used in weakness of stomach.

Used in joint pain and back pain.

It is useful in sciatica.

Effective in asthma.

To prevent phlegmatic diseases.

Useful in leprosy, Syphilis and leucoderma.

Used in all types of fevers periodic as well as chronic.

Used in Impotency, loss of sexual drive related drugs.

It is used in skin disease related ointment because of its corrosive nature.

Used in piles.

Mechanism of action: Antiseptic and siccative properties of processed arsenic is the reason of its blood purifaction activity.

Dose:15 mg to 30 mg with milk or butter.

Mode of Use:

Processed arsenic used in general weakness, nerve weakness, loss of libido, anemia, erythrocytopenia, nerve diseases and phlegmatic diseases such as migraine, sciatica, paralysis, facial paralysis, asthma.

Arsenic is blood purifier in action so it is used in skin diseases such as syphilis, leprosy and leucoderma.

Arsenic is antipyretic in nature so used in periodic fever as well as chronic fever.

Due to its corrosive nature it is used in ointment.

Arsenic is used as *tila* in case of piles.

Some preventive measures are required as arsenic rapidly absorbed in blood such as –

Do not use empty stomach.

It is necessary to use it along with *Ghee.*

It is better to use in winter season.

Do not use in hot and severe diseases.

Research studies:

Following preclinical and clinical evidence shows that arsenic trioxide inhibits growth and promotes apoptosis in many different cancer cell types.

Priclnical:

Myeloid leukemia, Myeloma,

Prostate cancer cell lines, Cervical cancer cell line,

Bladder cancer cell lines, Gastric cancer cell line,

Esophageal cancer cell line,

Clinical:

Hematologic malignancy, Advanced hormone-refractory prostate cancer, Advanced renal cell cancer, Advanced cervical cancer, Refractory transitional cell carcinoma of the bladder, proconvulsant activity

Toxicity: Fatal

Correctives: Milk, Ghee

Substitute: Hartal

Compound formulations: Kushtajat, kushta faulad, Kushta Sankhya, Johar seen, Johar raskapoor, Johar kala, Habbe Falij, Habbe ahmar, Tila jaded, Tila Surkh

SARPHUKA

Vernaculars

Arabic	:	Sarboka
Persian	:	Sufar
Urdu	:	Sarphoka
Hindi	:	Sarphenka, Sarphankha
English	:	Purple Tephrosia, Wild Indigo
Latin	:	Tephrosia purpurea Pers.
Family	:	Fabaceae

Introduction and History

Tephrosia purpurea Linn.(*T. purpurea*) is a well-known plant described in the ancient text of Unani meaning "*ash-colored*," referring to the grayish tint given to the leaves. It belongs to high medicinally valued plant family Fabaceae, comprising of more than 400 species. It has a long history of its use as an important drug for the treatment of syphilis, gonorrhea, leprosy and various skin diseases.

Habit and Habitat:

It's a perennial erect or decumbent herbs or subshrubs, up to 50 cm tall. is found throughout India and Sri Lanka flourishing in poor soil, through the plains of India, Ceylon, Mauritius, Tropical Africa and subtropical regions.

Description in Unani:

The morphological characteristics of Sarphuka in Unani literature is not as efficient as needed for its identification. However, some of the key features are described by some Unani physicians, on the basis of that description Sarphuka is identified as the plant of *Tephrosia purpurea* Linn. According to Unani literature Sarphuka is an Indian origin plant, half meter long, stem is thin has many branches, leaves are arranged in parallel manner. It bears flowers and legumes.

Its two types are mentioned on the basis of colour of the flower. One has white flowers and other has red flowers. The plants bearing white flowers are rare. Seeds are small kidney shaped, four to five seeds are found in a single pod. Taste of whole plant is bitter and unpleasant.

Botanical description:

T. purpurea is a perennials, erect or decumbent herbs or sub shrubs, height ranges from 50 cm to 1.5 meter. Compound leaves imparipinnate; terminal leaflets 7-15, 1-2.8 x 0.3-1 cm, oblanceolate or obovate, base cuneate, apex obtuse toemarginate. Flowers 7 mm long, purplish to white, bisexual, symmetrically, zygomorphic, hypogynous. In few-flowered, leaf is opposed, pseudoracemes; pedicels 3-4 mm long; bracts, 2 mm long, calyx, 3-4 mm long. Corolla, pink to purplish; 4 mm broad, orbicular and staminal tube, 4 mm long. Pod is dry dehiscent 2.5-4 x 0.3-0.4 cm, linear-oblong, 5-7-seeded. Seeds are ellipsoid, dark brown in colour.

Parts used: roots, leaves, seeds and stem bark

Chemical constituents:

The leaves contain rutin and rotenoids 0.65-0.80 % on dry basis). Rotenoid content is highest in the seed (1.60-1.80%). The leaves also contain a triterpenoid, lupeol, and beta-sitosterol. Seeds contain a diketone-pongamol; a dimethylchromene flavanone isolonchocarpin; furanoflavones karanjin and kanjone; a flavanone purpurin; and sitosterol. A flavonoid, lanceolarin B, is also present in seeds. The plant extract led to marked lowering of blood glucose level in normal and alloxan-induced diabetic rabbits. In diabetic rabbits the extract exerted 620-70 % hypoglycaemic effect as compared to tolbutamide. Shveta Sharapunkhaa (stems: covered withwhite hair; flowers: pale pink or pale violet) is equated with *T. villosa* Pers.The roots gave a prenylated flavanone 7-methylglabranin; pods contain rotenoids—villosin, villon, villosol, villosinol, villinol and villosone. The fresh root is credited with hypoglycaemic properties, but leaves did not.

Mizaj: hot and wet in first degree

Pharmacological actions: blood purifier, diuretic, antidote, anthelmintic, antipyretic, tonic, laxative, deobstruent, digestive, euphoretic and antileprotic properties.

Unani mechanism of action:

T. purpurea is one such drug which is listed in the blood purifier group of drugs. It has the property to purify blood from toxic substances by various mechanisms. Since its taste is bitter and temperament is hot therefore it has a number of pharmacological properties viz. demulcent, laxative, resolvent, deobstruent, diuretic, antiseptic etc. By virtue of these characteristics it is able to transform the morbid viscous matter into such a form which can be easily evacuated by the body. Since it has laxative and diuretic property therefore morbid matters are removed by respective organs. It also has the property to tone up the function of sluggish liver, kidney and stomach, in this way it does not only cure the disease but also prevent it by normalizing the performance of all these organs.

Therapeutic uses:

In the light of above mechanism of action, *T. purpurea* is used in the treatment of all those diseases which are caused by impure/ morbid blood such as acne, ulcer, itching, leprosy, syphilis, fever, inflammation and numerous skin disorders as well as venereal diseases. Since each part of *T. purpurea* has medicinal properties therefore either whole plant or its part are used in the treatment of various disorders e.g. Tender leaves have good results in treating eczema and vitiligo or patchy skin. It is also used to reduce blood toxicity caused by heavy metallic drugs or bhasma. Apart from skin diseases Sarphuka is also used in various other ailments of the body. For this purpose, it is either used orally in various dosage forms viz. powder, syrup, decoction, extract, tablet etc. or locally as paste and ointment. Its root is diuretic, allays thirst and enriches blood. The dried herb is given for the treatment of bronchitis, bilious febrile attacks, boils, pimples and bleeding piles. The leaf decoction is used for treating fever, heart and spleen disorders, digestive complaints, asthma and cancerous tumors. The extract of leaf is used in the management of abortion, quaternary and tertiary fever. Apart from single and compound formulations, *Sarphuka* is also combined with other drugs viz.100 gm of crushed leaves of *Sarphuka* and 50gm of cannabis leaves (*Cannabis sativa* Linn.) are mixed together, from which 4-6 gm if taken regularly for forty days cures piles. Tablet made from black pepper (*Piper nigrum)* and fresh root of *Sarphuka,* is used to reduce chronic gastric problems. If the paste of black pepper (5gm) and *Sarphuka* (7gm) applied locally reduces the inflammation of breast. Juice of *Sarphuka* with dry ginger (*Zingiber officinale* Roscoe.) provides relief from irritable bowel syndrome and with clove (*Syzygium aromaticum*) powder relieves chronic diarrhoea. If used in combination with *baubadang* (*Embelia ribes*), is very useful in expelling intestinal worms. Leaves juice is effective in leprosy. It relieves constipation and effective in spleenomegaly.

Dose: 5 to 7 gm

Mode of Use: orally

Research Studies:

Analgesic and Anti-inflammatory activity, Anthelmintic activity, Anti hyperlipidemic activity, Anti pyretic activity, Antidiabetic activity, Antiepileptic Activity, Antileishmanial Activity, Antimalarial activity, Antimicrobial activity,

Antioxidant activity, Antiulcer activity, Antiviral activity, Anxiolytic activity,

CNS depressant and analgesic activity, Cytotoxic activity, Hepatoprotective activity, Mast cell stabilizing potential (anti allergic) activity, Nephroprotective and anti lithiatic activity, Spasmolytic, bronchodilator and vasorelaxant activity, Wound healing activity.

Toxicity: Unani physicians have not discussed any toxic effect of *T. purpurea,* however some of the physicians reported that it causes eructation.

Corrective: Brahmadandi (*Tricholepis glaberrima* DC)

Substitutes: Mundi *(Sphaeranthus Indicus)* or Neelkanthi (*Ajuga bracteosa*).

Compound formulations: *Sharbate musaffi, Safoof juzam, Arq maul jubn, Arq murakkab musaffie khun banushka kala.*

Seemab

Vernaculars

Arabic	:	Zaibaq
Hindi	:	Paara
English	:	Mercury
Persian	:	Seemab
Sanskrit	:	Ras raaj
Latin	:	Hydrargyrum

Introduction and History

Mercury is silver like shiny metal which is known to humans from very old period. It is useful in many diseases. But its high quantity is poisonous for individual.

Description in Unani:

It's a white liquid metal similar in appearance with melted silver. Heavier than other metals.

Description:

Mercury is a metal which is in liquid form at room temperature. It is silvery in appearance. It is the heaviest metal. About thirteen times heavier than water. Its boiling point is 660 C and at 690 C it converts into vapour state. It is insipid in taste. Mercury is insoluble in water. It is usually not found in pure form instead found in combination with other elements like gold, silver, sulphur etc. It is used after purification.

Mizaj: Cold second degree Wet third degree. According to many hot and wet (more appropiate)

Pharmacological actions:

Cicatrizant, blood purifier, aphrodisiac, avoricious, mughallize mani, general tonic, antiseptic, resolves phlegmatic diseases, vermicide.

Therapeutic uses:

Used in phlegmatic and brain diseases, Arthritis, Asthma, Bells palsy, Fluidity of semen, General weakness, Head lice, Leprosy, Paralysis, Pre mature ejaculation, Pruritis, Rhinitis, Sexual debility, Spasm, Syphilis, Tremor, Tuberculosis.

Mechanism of action: antiseptic and due to good resolavent of impure phlegm it purifies and cleans blood.

Mode of use:

Externally used in ointment for non-healing wound. lice, syphilis and skin diseases, etc.

Research studies:

Anti anxiety effects: The effects of cinnabar on anxiety-like behaviors in mice were studied using the elevated plus maze test. Cinnabar at the oral dose of 50 and 100 mg/kg/d for 10 days significantly improved the performance in the elevated maze test.

Sedative or hypnotic effects: Induction of renal metallothionein

Dose: In calcinated and purified form 15-30 mg

Toxicity: Toxic to mouth, throat, Stomach

Corrective: Milk, Ghee

Substitutes: Raanga Muklas

Compound formulations: Habbe siyah, Marhame Gulabi, Habbe Qoobah.

SHAITRA

Vernaculars		
Arabic	:	Baglatulmulk, Bukslatulmulik, Shahatraja
Persian	:	Shahatra, Shatara
Urdu	:	Shahatra
Hindi	:	Parpata
English	:	Fumitory
Latin	:	Fumaria parviflora Lam.
Syn.	:	*Fumaria officinalis* Linn., *Fumaria indica* lam.
Family	:	Fumariaceae

Introduction and History

According to wealth of India, Indian plant bearing the name "Shahtrah" or "Pitpapra" has been wrongly referred as *Fumaria officinalis* Linn. or *Fumaria paviflora* lam. by many authors, which are common fumitory in Europe but not found in India.

Habit and Habitat:

The *Fumaria* is a genus of herbs distributed in Asia, Europe and Africa. The *F. indica* plants are distributed over the greater part of India upto 438 m on the Himalayas, Baluchistan, Afganistan, Persia, and Mongolia. In Unani system of medicine it is used either as a single drug or as an ingredient in many of the Unani formulations which are used in treatment of various ailments of the body.

Description in Unani:

According to Unani physician plant is 6 inch in height, delicate, whitish in colour. Leaves are similar to carrot or coriander leaves. Flower is small and white in colour. Fruits are small, shiny and fresh fruits are bluish in colour. Taste is bitter. Shahtra found all over India in wheat and barley farm in winter season.

Botanical description: *F. indica* is a much-branched, suberect or diffuse, pale-green, annual herb. Leaves are multifid and more or less glaucous; leaflets are 2-4 in number and pinnatisect; segment is long, linear or linear-oblong, flat, and acute. Recemes have 10-12 flowers that are rather dense; bracts lanceolate-subulate and slightly acuminate, and pedicels (2.0-2.5 in number) are rarely 4.5 mm long, erect and thickened at the apex. Sepals are about 1.5 mm long, 0.5-1.0 mm broad, lanceolate or ovate, acuminate, more or less inciso-dentate, rose colored and often persistent in the young fruit. Corrola is 5-6 mm long and rose colored. Fruit is about 2.5 mm broad, subrotund, quadrate, subtruncate and sometimes obscurely retuse. Stem is light green, smooth, hollow, about 3-4 mm thick, with root brown color and branches that are about 2-3 mm thick, and cylindrical.

Parts used: seeds and leaves

Chemical constituents:

Phytoconstituents present in different parts of *F. indica*.

Aerial part: Papracine, paprazine, sitosterol, stigmasterol, campesterol

Root: Protopine, octacosanol, narceimine, narlumidine, adlumidine

Leaf & stem: Narlumicine, protopine, narlumidine, nona cosanol

Seed : Fumariline, tetrahydrocoptisine, bicuculine, oxysanguinarine

Mizaj: hot and dry in second degree

Pharmacological actions:

Appetizer, Astringent, Blood purifier, Decreases the viscosity of blood. Deobstruent, Desiccant, Detergent, Diuretic, Gastro protective, Tonic to eye, Tonic to stomach,

Root bark: deobstruent, appetizer, blood purifier, stomach and liver tonic, antipyretic, diuretic.

Unani mechanism of action:

Because of bitterness, deobstruent, detergent properties, it removes abnormal *sawda,* it decreases viscosity of blood hence decreases heat of blood. It cleans blood from bilious toxins which leads to coldness in blood.

Therapeutic uses:

Chronic Fever, Jaundice, Joint pain, Leprosy, Obstruction of Liver and Spleen, Pain on other parts of body, Pruritus, Ring worm, Saudawi Diseases, Scabies, Septic Blood, Syphillis, Nausesa.

Dose: 5-7 g

Mode of Use:

Fresh leaves application is beneficial on insect biting.

If crushed with *mehandi* leaves relives itching.

Application of juice on eye improves eyesight.

Rinsing with its joshanda gives strength to gums and heals ulcers of mouth.

Internally leaves of shaitra stops nausea and vomiting and with *haleela zard* it increases appetite.

If used with alcohol is gives strength to stomach.

If used with vinegar increases appetite

Its juices when drinks with milk and jaggery treat the heat of stomach.

Drinking joshanda treats jaundice and bilious fever.

If its juice is drink with jaggery helps in removing toxins of the body, saudawi diseases, itching and fungal infection.

Decoction of Shahtra and Giloy cures seasonal fever.

Research Studies:

Anthelmintic activity, Antibacterial activity, Antidiabetic activity, Anti-eczema activity, Antifeedant activity, Anti-inflammatory activity, Antimicrobial activity, Antinociceptive activity, Antioxidant activity, Antiparasitic activity, Antiprotozoal activity, Antipruritic activity, Gastrointestinal activity, Hepatoprotective activity.

Toxicity: Lungs

Corrective: Tukhme Kasni

Substitutes: Haleela Zard

Compound formulations: Itrifal Shahatra, Arq–e-Shahtra

Sheesham

Vernaculars

Arabic	:	sasam
Persian	:	shesham pausaat
Urdu	:	Sheesham
Hindi	:	Shisham, sissu, sissai, sisam
English	:	Indian Rosewood, Bombay blackwood
Latin	:	Dalbergia sissoo DC.
Family	:	Fabaceae

Introduction and History

Dalbergia sissoo is a major genus of the woody legumes and belongs to the family Fabaceae (old Leguminosae), order Fabales (Shakya and Lakhey, 2007). It grows abundantly and forms a forest. s. It's adaptability, drought resistance, hardiness and nitrogen fixing properties, as well as its multipurpose nature makes it suitable for afforestation and reforestation programs in many parts of the country.

Habit and Habitat

Dalbergia sissoo is found in tropical to subtropical climates in natural and planted forests, very widely distributed in Pakistan, India, Afghanistan, Persia, Iraq, Kenya and Tanzania.

Description in Unani:

Sheehsam is a well known tree of India seen near river. Size of tree is approximately 60 feet. Leaves are small pointed. pods arranged in bunches. Each pod contains two to three seeds. Heart wood sap is about 1 inch thick. Yellowish in color.

Botanical description: Dalbergia sissoo DC is a medium to large tree of about 25 meters high with grey-yellow trunk, longitudinal crack, and downcast twig. Leaves are leathery, pinnately compound, with about five alternate leaflets. Leaf stalk (petiole) measures about 15 cm long, each leaflet widest at the base, to 6 cm long with a fine pointed tip. Flowers are whitish to pink, fragrant, nearly sessile, up to 1.5 cm (0.59 in) long and in dense clusters 5–10 cm (2.0–3.9 in) in length. Pods are oblong, flat, thin, strap-like 4–8 cm (1.6–3.1 in) long, 1 cm (0.39 in) wide and light brown. They contain 1–5 flat bean-shaped seeds 8–10 mm (0.31–0.39 in) long.

Parts used: heartwood

Chemical constituents:

Leaves: Isoflavone-O-glycoside. Flowers: Biochenin A, tectorigenin, 7, 4dimethyle tectorigenin and 7-O- methyle tectorigenin. Green pods: Mesoinisitol, 7-O- methyle tectorigenin and 4'-rhamnoglucoside. Mature pods: Isocaviumin, tectorigenin, dalbergin, caviunin and tannins. Stem bark: Dalberginone, dalbergin, methyl dalbergin and dalbergichromene. Heartwood: Dalbergin, nordalberginones, dalbergichromene, fixid oil and essential oils.

Mizaj: hot dry first degree

Pharmacological actions:

Abortificiant, Anti obesity, Antihelmenthic, Blood Purifier, Desiccant, Digestive.

Unani mechanism of action:

Bitter taste, digestive and dessicant propoerties confined its blood purification action.

Therapeutic uses:

Blood disorders, Boils, Burning sensations, Cutaneous diseases, Eruptions, Eye and nose disorders, Intestinal worms, Leprosy, Nausea, Obesity, Scabies, scalding urine, Spermatorrhea, Stomach problems, Stomatitis, Syphillis, Vitiligo.

Dose: 5 to 10 gm

Mode of Use:

bean with catechu is beneficial in mouth sores.

Decoction of leaves cures different skin problems and stops vomiting.

Decoction of leaves or wood is useful in leprosy.

Local application of leaves is useful in shoe bite, wound, burning skin etc.

Washing hairs with leaves of sheesham strengthens the hair.

Buds of sheesham with red chili used in Psychological diseases.

Research Studies

Antidiabetic effect, Antidiarrhoeal effect, Antiinflammatory and analgesic effects,

Antimicrobial effect, Antioxidant effect, Antiparasitic effect, Antiulcer effect, Cardiac effect, Dermatological effects, Memory booster, Osteogenic effects, Reproductive effect.

Toxicity: Hot Temperament

Corrective: Gond babul/ honey

Substitutes: Aabnus

Compound formulations: Sharbat Sheesham

Unnab

Vernaculars

Arabic	:	Unnaab
Persian	:	Kunar, Selanah
Urdu	:	Unnab
Hindi	:	Baer, Ber, Beri
English	:	Jujube Fruit, Chinese date
Latin	:	Ziziphus jujuba Mill.
Family	:	Rhamnaceae

Introduction and History

Ziziphus jujuba Mill. (*Z. jujuba*) is a traditional herb with a long history of use for nutrition and the treatment of a broad spectrum of diseases. It grows mostly in South and East Asia, as well as in Australia and Europe.

Habit and Habitat:

Lebanon, Iran, Pakistan, India, Bangladesh, Nepal, the Korean peninsula, south-eastern Europe and, southern and central China.

Description in Unani:

Botanical description:

Ibn Sina in his book Al Qanoon fil Tib mention that Unnab are the fruits. According to Najmul Ghani, Unnab are the fruits of a tree resembling ber, it is red colored and sweet to taste. Ibn Baithar in his book mentions that Unnab is the fruit of a tree, which are red colored and sweet to taste having nutritional and medicinal values.

Parts used: Fruits, leaves, bark, gum

Chemical constituents: Research shows that jujube fruits are rich in the phenolic compounds catechin and rutin. The jujube fruit has high sugar content and high levels of vitamin A, C and B complexes, vitamin E, phosphorus and calcium).

Mizaj: Cold, Hot moist, Motadil

Pharmacological actions:

Fruits: Blood purifier, expectorant, laxative, anti scabies, demulcent of humours, sedative to heat of bilioius and sanguineous humours, aperients for thoracic region, etc

Leaves: antipyretic, laxative

Seeds: hypnotic, sedative, stomach tonic

Unani mechanism of action: Unnab purifies the blood hence used in many of the compound formulations of blood purifiers. It decreases the viscosity of *khilt and* Removes raqeeq through intestine. It increases the Production of clean blood. According to Avicenna it decreases the heat of bilioius and sanguineous humours.

Therapeutic uses:

Acne, Blood disease, Boils pustules, Catarrh, Cough, Itching, Measles, Periodic fever, Pharyngitis, Pleurisy, Pneumonia, Pyrexia, Seasonal fever, Skin diseases, Small pox, Syphilis.

Dose: 5 to 7 fruit

Mode of Use*:*

Unnab (fruit) relieves thirst and is beneficial in constipation. Chewing of the unnab leaves reduces nausea. Powdered seeds of unnab causes constipation, hence used in diarrhoea. It is also used in diseases of rectum. Jujube is used prophylactically for liver diseases. The fruits are also used in Chinese medicine to strengthen liver function.

Unnab is used in sozish masana (cystitis).

Its joshanda (decoction) and khaisanda is beneficial in dry cough and dryness of throat.

Chewing of the Unnab leaves has anesthetic effect in the throat and tongue.

Powdered bark of Unnab with equal quantity of Safeda is beneficial in non healing ulcers and 200 ml Joshanda of leaves of Unnab with sugar is beneficial in itching. Unnab with arq kasni and sikanjabeen is beneficial in small pox.

Research Studies:

Antiallergic, anti-anaphylactic activity, Antibacterial Activity, Anti-cancer activity of *Ennab*, Antidiabetic, Antifertility/ contraceptive property, Antioxidants, Antimicrobial and Anti-inflammatory, Antispastic effect, Cognitive activities, Hepatoprotective activity, Hypotensive and Antinephritic effect, Immuno-stimulant effects, Permeability enhancement activity, Sedative activity, Sweetness inhibitors, Wound healing activity.

Toxicity: Stomach

Corrective: Rose, honey, sugar

Substitutes: sapisatan

Compound formulations:

Sharbat Unanb, Sharbat Aejaz, Lauq Sapistan, Khameera gaozaban sheera unnabwala, Sharbat sadar, Sharbat murakkab musaffie khun, Itrifal zamani

USHBA

Vernaculars

Arabic	:	Ushba
Persian	:	Ushba Maghrabi
Urdu	:	Ushba
Hindi	:	Ushva
English	:	Mexican Sarsaparilla
Latin	:	*Smilax aristolochiaefolia*
Family	:	Liliaceae

Introduction and History

The drug Ushba consists of dried roots of *Smilax aristolociaefolia* Mill. the plant a climber; native to America, Mexico and the West Indies.

The French physician Monardes described using sarsaparilla to treat syphilis in 1574. In 1812, Portuguese soldiers suffering from syphilis recovered faster if sarsaparilla was taken to treat the disease versus mercury, the standard treatment at the time.

It is important to know that H. indicus is referred to as Indian sarsaparilla and it is used as substitute for sarsaparilla, Smilax aristolochiaefolia and their 26 species and varied of family Smilacaceae. It is employed as a vehicle for potassium iodide and for purposes for which sarsaparilla is used. In India it is employed as a substitute for that substance as an alterative, tonic, diuretic and diaphoretic.

Habit and Habitat:

Ushba is common in wooded areas because it uses its tendrils to climb up the trees. It is widely found in temperate, swampy and warm areas. Sarsaparilla is also found in high elevations; in Nuevo León, Mexico, it is found at elevation of 1760 meters, in Oaxaca at 100 meters, in Hacienda San Jose, Santa Ana at 850 to 1100 meters

Description in Unani:

According to Ram Lubhaya it's climber with tendrils. It has thin, venated cylindrical root and stem slightly reddish in color bitter in taste. Many authors consider Ushba as foreign Anantmol. In India this plant is imported from abroad particularly America. Flower is white and arranged in bunches, leaves are broad. In Indian Ushba is found in south region, kalkaji. Taste is sweetish and acrid and odourless.

Botanical description:

The roots are narrow, very long, cylindrical, upto 6mm in diameter and usually found in commerce folded and bound into bundles; pieces of rhizome present which is much thicker; external surface of the root varies from grayish to reddish brown, longitudinally wrinkled, occasionally smooth, fracture short or tough and fibrous in the central cylinder, taste sweetish and acrid and odourless.

Parts used: Root

Chemical constituents: Acetyl-parigenin, astilbin, â-sitosterol, dihydroquercetin, diosgenin, epsilon-sitosterol, eucryphin, ferulic acid, kaemferol, parillin, saponin, sarasaponin, smilagenin and stigmasterol.

Mizaj: Hot and Dry third degree/second degree

Pharmacological actions:

Alterative, Analgesic, Anti inflammatory, Blood purifier, Demulcent, Diaphoretic, Diuretic, carminative

Unani mechanism of action: Blood purifying properties is due to its muarriq, muraqqiq and mulattif action.

Therapeutic uses:

Ascites, Arthririts, Kidney pain, Balghami diseases, Chronic skin diseases, Cough, Facial palsy, Leprosy, Melasma/cholasma, Paralysis, Pruritus, Syphilis, Tremor.

Dose: 7 gm

Mode of Use:

Ushba 70 gm, saung 10 gm, bisfaij 30 gm, turbud 10 gm, honey 750 gm and sugar 750 gm add all theses ingredient and make Majun. This majun is very effective in syphillis, cleaning urinary tract, pruritus and eczema, joint pain, insomnia and various saudawi diseases.

Orally Powder of Ushba is effective in chronic cough, ascities, piles and sciatica. Locallyit helps in wound healing.

Research Studies:

Adjuvant for the treatment of leprosy, Anti-inflammatory, Diuretic, Hematopoetic activity, Hepatoprotective, Improvement in psoriasis, Improvement of appetite and digestion, Hypoglycemic, hypotensive.

Toxicity: Hot temperament

Corrective: Almond oil

Substitutes: China root

Compound formulations: Majoon-e-Ushba, Arq ushba, Naqu shatra

Compound formulation:

Followings are some compound drugs havingblood puririfer properties.

Arq Mundi

Mundi 250 gm
Water 6 liter

Action: musaffie dam, muqawwi basar

Use: Zofe basar, Fasade dam

Dose: 75 to 100 ml orally

Arq Murakkab Mussafi Khūn

Burada abnus 50 gm
Burada sheesham 50 gm
Burada sandal sukrh 50 gm
Burada sandal safaid 50 gm
Barge heena 50 gm
Barge neem 250 gm
Barhamdandi 50 gm
Post haleela zard 50 gm
Chiraita tallkh 50 gm
Sarphooka 50 gm
Shaitra 50 gm
Unnab 50 gm
Gule Mundi 50 gm
Gule Niloofar 50 gm
Haleela Siyah 50 gm
Water 8 litre

Action: Musaffie khoon

Uses: Fasade Dam, Itching, Boils, Abscess, Gonorrhea, Syphilis

Dose: 125 ml orally with Sharbat Unnab

Arq Shahtra

Shahtra 850 gm
Water 12 litre

Action: blood purifier

Uses: Fasade dam, Joint pain

Dose: 75 ml

ARQ USHBA

Chob chini 125 gm
Ushba maghrabi 62.5 gm
Anant mol 187.5 gm
Water 8 litre

Action: blood purifier

Uses: fasade khoon, joint pain

Dose: 75 ml od with sharbat Unnab.

Habbe Daad

Suhaga 25 gm
Gandhak 25 gm
Neela Toothiya 25 gm
Paara 25 gm
Abe lemon 40 ml

Action: Blood purifier

Uses: Ringworm

Doses: Rub one tablet in lemon water and apply local.

HABBE KATH

Kafoor 10

Raskapoor 10

Kathsafaid 10

Musli safaid 20

Aabe barge tambool.50

Action: Mubarrid, dafe, taffun, musaffi

Uses: Aatishk

Dose: 250 to 500 mg

Habb-e-Musaffi-e-Khoon

Berg Bakayin 10 g

Berg Neem 10 g.

Berg Hina 30 g

Burada Sandal Surkh 30 g

Barham Dandi 30 g

Post Halela Zard 30 g

Chaksu 30 g

Rasaut 30 g

Zeera Safaid 10 g

Sarphoka 30 g

Sahtara 30 g

Filfil Siyah 10 g

Kishneez Khushk 30 g

Post Kachnal 10 g

Gul-e-Surkh 30 g

Neel Kanthi 30 g

Action: Musaffi-e-Khoon and Habis ud Dam

Therapeutic Use: In Nazf ud Dam

Dose: Children: One to two pills (each 80 mg.)

Adult: Four Pills

Itrifal Mundi

Post haleela zard 120 gm
Haleela siyah 120 gm
Post haleela kabuli 120 gm
Post baleela 120 gm
Aamla khushk 120 gm
Tukhme kishneez 120 gm
Barge shaitra 120 gm
Aslussoos 120 gm
Ustukhudus 120 gm
Gule mundi 80 gm
Qand safaid 3 kg
Raughan zard Q.S

Action: Musafiie dam

Uses: Fasade dam, ring worm, ramad

Dose: 10 to 20 gm

Itrifal Shahtra

Aamla 100 gm
Post Baleela 100 gm
Post haleela zard 350 gm
Sana 50 gm
Shaitra 250 gm
Gule surkh 30 gm
Ghee 120 gm
Mawaz munaqqa 350 gm
Shakar safaid 2 kg 650 gm
Satte lemon 3gm

Action: Musaffie dam

Uses: Syphilis, itching, fasade khoon

Dose: 5 to 10 gm BD with 60 ml of water

Majun Chob Chini

Ilaichi khurd 50 gm
Andarjosheeren 50 gm
Bozidan 50 gm
Peepal kala 20 gm
Javitri 10 gm
Jadwar 20 gm
Jaiphal 10 gm
Chob chini 300 gm
Khulanjan 10 gm
Daarchini 5 gm
Zaranbad 10 gm
Zanjabeel 20 gm
Saad kufi 10 gm
Sana 50 gm
Suranjan shereen 50 gm
Aqar qarha 20 gm
filfil siyah 50 gm
Qaranfal 10 gm
Gule surkh 10 gm
Sugar 2.5 kg
Zafran1.80 gm
Arqe gauzaban 15 ml
Mastagi 40 gm
Ghee 10 gm

Action: Blood purifier

Uses: Joint pain, blood diseases

Dose : 6 gm bd

Majun Ushba

Amla 25 gm
Afteemun 300 gm
Anant mol 100 gm
Burada sandal surkh 50 gm
Burada sandal safaid 50 gm
Badiyan 100 gm
Balchad 50 gm
Bisfaij 100 gm
Balila 30 gm
Post halila zard 25 gm
Chob chini 50 gm
Darchini 50 gm
Sana makki 200 gm
Shaitra 50 gm
Ushba magribi 100 gm
Kabab chini 50 gm
Gule surkh 100 gm
Halila 25 gm
Sugar 4.6 kg

Action: mulayyin, blood purifier

Uses: Jarb, wajaul mufasil, hikka

Dose: 5 to 10 gm

Majun Mundi

Post halela zard 100 gm

Baleela 50 gm

Aamla 50 gm

Haleela siyah 50 gm

Kishniz khushk 50 gm

Shahtra 50 gm

Aslussos 50 gm

Gule mundi 400 gm

Qand safaid 3.5 kg

Ghee 50 gm

Aciton: Musaffie dam

Uses: fasad ud dam, ramad, itching, syphilis, gonorrhea, arthritis

Dose: 10 to 15 gm od with water

Majun Musaffi-e-Azam

Barg-e-Shahtara 200 g
Post Halela Zard 160 g
Post Halela Kabli 120 g
Post Balela 400 g
Aamla Khushk 400 g
Halela Siyah 300 g
Barg-e-Sana 50 g
Gul-e-Surkh 120 g
Maweez Munaqqa 1.5 Kg
Bisfayej Fistaqi 130 g
Aftimoon 130 g
Turbud 130 g
Qand Safaid 8 Kg

Action: Musaffi-e-Dam, Mukhrij-e-Mawad-e-Fasida

Therapeutic Use: Busoor, Damameel, Kharish, Aatishak, Waj-ul-Mafasil, Waram-e-Mafasil

Dose: 6 g with 50 ml Araq-e-Musaffi Murakkab or with water twice daily.

Majun Musaffi Khas

Aftimoon Wilayti 2g
Burada Sandal Surkh 1 g
Burada Sandal Safaid 1 g
Badiyan 10 g
Bisfayej 10 g
Balchhar 5 g
Post Halela Zard 2 g
Chob Chini 3 g
Darchini 5 g
Rewand Chini 5 g
Saqmonia Wilayti 5 g
Sana Makki 10 g
Anantmool 40 g
Kabab chini 5 g
Gul Surkh 10 g
Halela Siyah 5 g
Qand Safaid 400 g
Milah Firangi 5 g
Warq-e-Nuqra 1g

Action: Musaffi-e-Khoon

Therapeutic Use: In Fasad-e-khoon, Kharish, Aatishak and Suzak

Dose: 5 g.

Sharbat Murakkab Musaffie Khūn

Burada abnus 50 gm
Burada sheesham 50 gm
Burada sundal surkh 100 gm
Burada sandal safaid 50 gm
Beenkh oont katara 50 gm
Post haleela zard 50 gm
Sarphooka 50 gm
Shaitra 100 gm
Unnab 250 gm
Sugar 4 kg
Satte lemon 12 gm
Natroon banjawi 6 gm

Action: Musaffie

Uses: Fasade khoon, Syphillis, itching, Ringworm etc.

Dose : 25 ml bd with arq murakkab musaffie khun or water.

Sharbat Unnab

Unnab 600 gm

Water 4 litre

Qand Safaid 4kg

Satte lemon 120 gm

Natrun banjawi 6 gm

Action: Musakkin, Munaffis

Use: Cough, skin diseases

Dose: 20 to 60 ml

Patent Products: Following are some patenet regsiterd products of pharmaceutical companies

Safi (Hamdard)

Each 5 ml content

Sana 160.45 mg

turbud 25.45 mg

Gulab ka phul 24.77 mg

Burada sheesham 13.40 mg

Sandal surkh 11.36 mg

Gilo 14.09 mg

Harar 22.04 mg

Narkachoor 11.36 mg

Chiraita 17.38 mg

Kasaundi 13.40 mg

Mundi 15.45 mg

Nilkanthi 16.13 mg

Shahtra 22.72 mg

Kachnal 15.45 mg

Neem 19.43 mg

Tulsi 13.40 mg

Zaranbaad 11.36 mg

Dar hald 9.43 mg

Chob chini 11.36 mg

Post keekar 42.80 mg

Sankhaholi 14.09 mg

Sarphooka 18.06 mg

Ushba 5.68 mg m

Brahmi 9.09 mg

Chaksu 9.09 mg

Beekh kasni 9.09 mg

Unnab 11.36 mg

Rewand chini 22.72 mg

Qand safaid

Shora desi 227.27 mg

Mileh firangi 1.25 gm

Action:

Anthelmintic: Expel parasitic worms (helminths) and other internal parasites from the body.

Anti–inflammatory: Reducing inflammation by acting on body mechanisms.

Antioxidant: Neutralize the oxidant effect of free radicals and other substances.

Antibacterial: Active against bacteria.

Anti–viral: Effective against viruses.

Carminative: Preventing the formation or causing the expulsion of flatulence.

Diuretic: Promoting excretion of urine/agent that increases the amount of urine excreted.

Depurative: Purifying agent.

Detoxifying: remove toxic substances.

Digestive: Digestant.

Purgative: laxative in effect.

Uses: skin diseases, poor immunity, worm infestation, viral infection etc.

Dose: 10 ml for adults 5 ml for children two times a day

Rakt Safa (Dehalvi Remedies)

Each 10 ml contains

Brahm dandi 200 mg

Barge neem 200 mg

Chiraita talkh 200 mg

Chob chjini 200 mg

Gule surkh 100 mg

Halela siyah 200 mg

Halela zard 200 mg

Jawansa 100 mg

Kamila surkh 100 mg

Gule mundi 200 mg

Zaranbad 200 mg

Neel kanthi 200 mg

Post bakain 200 mg

Post neem 200 mg

Sandal surkh 200 mg

Sandal safaid 100 mg

Sarphooka 200 mg

Shahtra 200 mg

Unnab 400 mg

Ushba maghrabi 100 mg

Sugar (ext) 10 ml

Action: blood purifier

Uses: blood impurities, boils, carbuncles, impetigo, pimples scroufula, seborrhea, acne, dermatitis, urninary irritation, prickly heat and itches, for improving skin complexion, skin diseases.

Dose: 10 ml in the morning with water

Musaffie Ajeeb (Rex)

Introduction

- Unani medicine that is used as a blood purifier
- Helps to correct the the digestive system and relieves constipation
- Prevents pimples and skin eruptions
- Reduces pigmentation and dark spots

Berge hina 25 mg
Barge bakain 200 mg
Barge neem 200 mg
Bisfaij 200 mg
Burada sheesham 100 mg
Barham dandi 200 mg
Chiraita 200 mg
Chobchini 200 mg
Darhald 100 mg
Gule surkh 100 mg
Gule mundi 175 mg
Halela zard 200 mg
Katehli 100 mg
Khas 200 mg
Nigandh babri 100 mg
Post neem 200 mg
Shahtra 200 mg
Sarphooka 200 mg
Sandal surkh 100 mg
Unnab 400 mg
Ushba maghrabi 100 mg

Zaranbaad 200 mg

Qand safaaid Q.S

Sodium benzoate Q.S

Action: Has anti-inflammatory, antibacterial, and antimicrobial properties, which help to reduce inflammation in the dermal layer of the skin.

Uses: Used in the treatment of acne vulgaris

It helps to reduce blemishes and dark spots

Dose: Musaffi Ajeeb should be taken in dosage of 2 teaspoons (10 ml) thrice daily for at least 4 weeks.

Lalima Bloob Purifier

Introduction

Zandu lalima contains natural ingredients with essence oil that helps to purify blood and skin and make skin pimple and acne free. It also promotes good blood circulation and provides nourishment to skin. Zandu Lalima Also Leads To A Pinkish Glow On The Face, Reduces Future Occurance Of Pimples To A Great Extent.

Each 5 ml (one teaspoonful)

Contains aqueous extracts of: Nimba 75 mg, Keshar 1 mg, Madhu (Honey) 0.1 gm, Godhum Te l(wheat germ oil) 5 mg, Bhringaraj 75 mg, Triphala 150 mg, Anantamool 150 mg, Haridra 150 mg, Manjistha 75 mg, Guduchi 75 mg, Katuki 60 mg, Chirata 60 mg Flavoured sugar syrup base & Preservatives (Methyl Paraben 0.1%, Propyl Paraben 0.02% & Sodium benzoate 0.5%) q.s. Essence: Menthol 1.0 mg, Camphor 3.0 mg, Spearmint Oil 3.75 mg. Excipients: Tween-80 10.0 mg, Citric Acid 1.25 mg.

Action: Blood purification and rejuvenation of skin

Uses:

- Helps to remove pimple, acne.
- Rejuvenate the skin.
- Provide Glow to skin.
- Dose Dosage everyday
- a blemish free long lasting pinkish fairness
- 2 tea spoon in an empty stomach with adequate amount of lukewarm water

Musaffein (Kiran Gandhi)

Ushba 2 gm
Neem 2 gm
Sarphooka 2 gm
Mundi 2 gm
Chaksu 2 gm
Bakain 2 gm
Neel kanthi 2 gm
Shaitra 2 gm
Sakhar safaid 60 gm

Action : blood purification

Uses: skin diseases

Dose: 6gm two times a day

MUSAFFEEN (NEW SHAMA)

Herbal blood purifier

Each dose of 10 ml contains aq extract of

Braham dandi 194 mg

Burada aabnoos 194 mg

Barge bakain 97 mg

Barge neem 97 mg

Ciraita talkh 194 mg

Chobchini 194 mg

Gule surkh 97 mg

Haleela siyah 194 mg

Haleela zard 194 mg

Hiran khuri 194 mg

Jawansa 94 mg

Kamila surkh 97 mg

Khus 194 mg

Gule mundi 194 mg

Neelkanthi 194 mg

Narkachoor 94 mg

Post neem 194 mg

Post bakain 194 mg

Barge shaitra 194 mg

Sarphuka 194 mg

Sandal surkh 194 mg

Sandal safaid 97 mg

Unnab 388 mg

Ushba 97 mg

Qand safaid 5.0 g

Aabe khaas qs

Preservative qs

Dose: Two tea spoonful in the morning and evening with water on empty stomach

Action: blood purification

Uses: acne, skin dullness

Khoon Safa (AMU Dawakhan)

Introducrion

AMU Dawakhana Khoon Safa is a special herbal product, which is prescribed to remove various impurities from the blood. It is mainly prescribed to people suffering from constipation and seasonal fever. It is a completely natural herbal remedy and is safe to use without causing any unwanted side effects.

Each dose of 10 ml content

Barge shahtra105 mg

Burada sandal safaid105 mg

Burada sandal surkh105 mg

Barge sana maki105 mg

Neel kanhti105 mg

Barham dandi105 mg

Burada sheesham105 mg

Gule mundi105 mg

Sarphooka105 mg

Nigand babri105 mg

Unnab105 mg

Post halela zard105 mg

Post halela siyah105 mg

Zaranbad105 mg

Gule surkh 105 mg

Kishneez kushk 105 mg

Barge neem 105 mg

Dare hald 105 mg

Chiraita talkh 105 mg

Barge hina 210 mg

Qand safaid

Action: A natural blood purifier, it rejuvenates the entire mechanism of the body

Khoon Safa cleanses all impurities from the blood

Uses: Purified blood is the most effective remedy for the treatment of skin disorders, such as pimples, boils, urticaria and associated issues

Useful in treating constipation and digestion-related issues

Dose: 10 ml adult, 5 ml children

Research Studies

4.1 Busoore labniya (Acne)

According to classical Unani literature it is described as common dermatological disorder of adolescent period manifest as white eruption over the face. According to Avicenna acne are small white eruptions on the nose and cheeks which resemble a drop of milk (Ibn Sina, 2007).

Efficacy of topical application of Safoofe Basoor - a polyherbal formulation

A randomized, single blind, standard controlled study was carried out on 60 patients. The test group was treated locally with formulation containing drugs *viz. Cinnamomum zeylanicum, Papaver somniferum* and *Euphorbia latex* while control group was treated with topical application of Tretinonin for a period of 8 weeks. The subject was assessed using Cook system of grading. The response of drug was recorded on a five point scale. The result showed that both the groups had significant effect ($p<0.001$) in ameliorating acne (Quamri *et al.*, 2009).

Effect of compound Unani formulation-Zimade Muhasa (ZM)

Another randomized, single-blind, standard controlled trial was conducted to evaluate the efficacy and tolerability of Unani topical anti acne formulation Zimade Muhasa against standard control (5% benzoyl peroxide) which was applied on Acne vulgaris on 48 patients. Content of test drug is *Iris germanica, Azadirachta indica, Abrus precatorius, Albizia lebbeck* and lake salt. After 6 weeks, both the treatment decreased the acne lesions significantly ($P<0.001$). Additionally, test drug significantly improved post inflammatory hyperpigmentation ($P<0.001$), scarring ($P=0.025$) and complexion ($P=0.001$). ZM was well-tolerated by patients and the efficacy was found to be equivalent to standard drug (Tabasum *et al.*, 2014).

Efficacy and safety of a polyherbal formulation

A standard controlled single blind clinical study on 50 patients of acne vulgaris was carried out. The formulation contains *Iris florentina, Azadirachta indica, Acacia speciosa, Abrus precatorious* and Lake Salt. Treatment duration was of 45 days and severity of acne vulgaris and efficacy of the drug was evaluated by employing Cook System of Acne Grading. Result demonstrated that herbal formulation and standard drug were equally effective and statistically significant ($p<0.05\%$). There was no significant difference in efficacy after treatment between the two groups at 5% p level. Further the Polyherbal formulation was found safe and fairly well accepted by the patients (Lone *et al.*, 2011).

Efficacy of Marhame Raal and Qurs Musaffie Khoon (Kit Medicine)

Sixty patients with active lesion of acne vulgaris were included in the open clinical trial to evaluate the efficacy of Unani kit medicine viz. Marham Raal (*Shorea robusta* resin, *Cinnamomum camphora, Acacia catechu,* oil of *Brassica nigra* and wax) and Qurs Musaffie Khoon (*Berberis artsiata, Zingiber zerumbet, Acacia catechu* and *Cassia absus*). The study shows that Marham Raal and Qurs Musaffie Khoon combination can be effective therapy in I, II and III grade acne vulgaris. In grade IV better results can be obtained if the duration of treatment is to be extended (Ara I, *et al.*, 2014).

Efficacy of local application of a Unani formulation in acne vulgaris

The study was observational self control (before and after treatment) on 40 female patients carried out for one year. *Nigella sativa, Ammonium chloride* and Būra Armani mixed with vinegar were applied locally for one month with low calorie index diet. All subjects were assessed on the basis of changes in objective and subjective parameters. The response of test formulation was found to be highly significant ($P<0.01$). Subjects reported a reduction of 82.6%, 80.9%, and 66.6% in tenderness, itching and irritation respectively (Sultana *et al.*, 2015).

4.2 Kalaf (Melasma)

Melasma is one of the common aesthetically displeasing entity continues to be a difficult problem to treat. According to Unani physicians it is caused by sub dermal oozing and accumulation of morbid blood or due to rupture of blood capillaries or congestion (Tabri, 1997).

Efficacy of Raphanus sativus and Apium graveolens with vinegar

A single blind, randomized and standard control, clinical study was conducted on 44 patients of melasma. *Apium graveolens* is a blood purifier (Tyagi *et al.*, 2013, Nilugal *et al.*, 2015). In test group ointment containing seeds of *Raphanus sativus* and *Apium graveolens* with vinegar was applied while in control group Azelaic acid, 10% cream was used for 45 days. Both the treatments were found to be equally effective (P= 0.001) in test and control group (Gauri *et al.*, 2015).

Efficacy of Nigella sativa and Sugarcane Vinegar

Another clinical study was done to find out the effect of a paste of *Nigella sativa* and vinegar on melasma. More than 75% improvement was observed in 50% cases and 50-75% improvement in 30% cases. No improvement was seen in 20% cases (Zarnigar *et al.*, 2011).

4.3 Bahaq (Pityriasis)

According to a renowned Unani Physician Rhazes (850-923 A.D.) pityriasis is a skin disease characterized by either hypo or hyper pigmentation with formation of scales on skin. Hakeem Ajmal Khan described pityriasis as an infectious or contagious disease characterized by white yellow patches on trunk and neck along with scaling of skin. It may or may not be associated with pruritus. HakeemAkbar Arzani (17th century A.D.) has classified pityriasis into two types, Bahaq Abyaz (white pityriasis) and Bahaq Aswad (Black pityriasis) (Arzani, 2002).

Efficacy of polyherbal ointment Zimade Bahaq containing *Plumbago zeylanica, Brassica nigra, Centipede minima, Rubia cordifolia, Raphanus sativus* and Vinegar.

A randomized, single-blind, standard controlled study was conducted on total 64 patients of Pityriasis. In test group Zimade Bahaq while in control group Sodium Thiosulphate Lotion (20 %) was applied for 30 days daily once. Study revealed that the efficacy of both the formulation is significant ($p<0.05$) but Unani formulation showed comparatively quicker response than the standard drug (Lone *et al.*, 2012).

4.4 Bars (Vitiligo)

Rhazes beautifully described pathophysiology of vitiligo. According to him when there is excessive accumulation of balgham ghaleez (thick phlegm) affected part becomes whitish and molluscs like. Further, the circulating blood is altered on reaching the affected part and becomes phlegmatic, and the area getting such blood cannot be nourished properly (Razi, 1991).

Efficacy of Safoof bars containing *Psoralea corylifolia, Cassia absus, Ficus hispida,* and *Cassia tora*

A randomized, single blind, placebo controlled study was undertaken to evaluate the efficacy of Safoofe Bars in the management of Vitiligo. The patient was divided in test (30 patients) and control group (10 patients). Duration of trial was 3 months with follow up of every 15 days. Response in test group was found to be statistically ($p<0.005$) significant (Ahmad *et al.*, 2011).

Therapeutic evaluation of compound formulation Majoon Atrilal along with local application of *Plumbago zeylanica* and Copper sulphate

An observational single blind study was carried out on 20 clinically diagnosed patients of vitiligo. They were given 10 gm of Majoon Atrilal twice daily along with local application of *Plumbago zeylanica* and Copper sulphate, daily once for three months. Vitiligo area study index showed significant improvement ($P<0.005$). Study revealed that these drugs are efficacious in vitiligo (Mohd *et al.*, 2014).

4.5 Shara (Urticaria)

According to Unani literature Urticaria is a disease which is caused by morbid blood. Excessive amount of safra (bile) or balgham shor (abnormal phlegm) may be the factors of such type of disorder. Severe heat of such blood causes abnormality in the nerves which ultimately result in urticaria rash (Tabri, 1997).

Therapeutic evaluation of local application of pearl shell and powder of *Rauwolfia serpentina*

A randomized, single-blind, placebo-controlled study was carried out on 30 patients (Test group included 20 patients and control group 10 patients). Test drug were given for 28 days twice daily. Results showed that the test drug produced significant ($p<0.05$) effect on itching, wheals, and erythema (Lone *et al.*, 2011).

Efficacy of polyherbal formulation prepared by *Rauvolfia serpentina, Acorus calamus, Artimisia vulgaris, Fumaria indica, Nardostachys jatamansi, Lavendula stoechas*

Unani formulation capsule Pitkriya containing above drugs were tested clinically for its efficacy and safety in the management of urticaria. Patient of urticaria were randomly assigned into two groups. Pitkriya treatment significantly decreased all the symptom score in patient of chronic urticaria. Statistically significant difference ($p\leq0.01$) was observed between two groups. The test formulation found to be safe, none of the values of haematological and biochemical parameters were outside normal range, and no clinically significant adverse effect was observed during and after 12 week of study (Shamsi *et al.*, 2006).

4.6 Qooba (Ring worm)

According to Unani physicians Ring worm is defined as type of roughness appears on the skin as a hyper pigmented patch having edge with itching and devoid of pain. This patch is usually circular in shape (Qarshi, 2011).

Assessment of local application of Marhame Qooba along with oral administration of Joshanda Mundi

The study was conducted as a single test drug Marhame Qooba for local application and Joshanda Mundi for oral administration for 60 days; while Tab. Fluconazole (150 mg orally and ointment Clotrimazole 1% for local application) were used as standard control for 30 days twice daily. The overall response in both the test and control groups was statistically significant ($p<0.05$) in the patients of ring worm. The study revealed that the test drug exhibited good response on itching, scaling and erythema (Mobeen *et al.*, 2012).

Efficacy of compound oral formulation Majoon Ushba and local application of Marham Gulabi

The efficacy of compound formulation Majoon Ushba and local application of Marham Gulabi was evaluated on 30 patients for a period of 45 days on the basis of improvement in the clinical subjective parameters like itching, scaling etc. The compound formulation had significant effect on itching (Hasan *et al.*, 2011).

4.7 Taqasshure Jild (Psoriasis)

Psoriasis is described in Unani literature under the caption "*Taqasshure jild*". Ancient Unani scholars Rofas, Galen, Rhazes, Avicenna, Majoosi, Avenzoar, Ibnul Qaf, and Ibne Hubul described it in detail. According to their description Psoriasisis a common skin disorder characterized by dryness of skin and scale formation like a fish (Qarshi, 2011).

Efficacy of local application of Roghane Hindi with orally used formulation, Majoon Ushba

A randomized, single blind, placebo controlled trial was done to assess the safety and efficacy of two pharmacopeial Unani formulations Majoon Ushba and Roghane Hindi in the management of psoriasis on scientific parameters. The duration of the trial was 8 weeks and follow-up was done fortnightly on thirty diagnosed psoriasis patients. The study demonstrated that these Unani formulations produce significant improvements ($P< 0.01$) in subjective and objective parameters (Lone *et al.*, 2011).

Therapeutic evaluation of a compound orally used formulation Itrifal Shahatra along with local application of Roghane Babchi

Another clinical study was designed to evaluate the efficacy of Unani Pharmacopoeal preparation Itrifal Shahatra and Roghane Babchi. Sixty patients were randomly selected and duration of study was 60 days. At the end of the study it was observed that there was improvement in erythema which was reduced up to 75%, burning sensation 100%, and over all well-being and improvement in disfigurement was statistically significant (Akhtar *et al.*, 2011).

Effect of Psoralia corylifolia with local application of Marhame Gulabi

The clinical study was conducted on 40 psoriatic patients. Patients were advised to take water of *Psoralia corylifolia* and apply Marhame Gulabi on the lesion once a day for 45 days. Clinical evidences proved the effectiveness of test drugs (Khan *et al.*, 2009).

4.8 Naarfaarsi (Eczema)

Eczema is a Greek word comprising two parts "Ec" means 'out' and "Zeo" means 'boil'. The whole word implies to "boil-out". The primary cause of Nar-e-Farsi (eczema) is production of excess quantity of abnormal safra (Yellow bile) mixed with abnormal sauda and sauda-e-muhtariqa (black bile). Therefore all the Unani physicians are of the opinion that its treatment should be started with tanqiyah-e-badan (removal of harmful material from the body) through different means of evacuation like fasd, munzij and mushil etc (Qarshi, 2011).

Efficacy of *Smilax china* with topical application of Murdar sang, Roghane gul, Safeda, Sirka and Kafoor

A randomized, single blind, placebo controlled study was conducted on total fifty patients to find out the efficacy of *Smilax china* with topical application of Unani formulation. *Smilax china* powder was administered orally along with topical application of ointment comprises of Murdar sang (Litharge), Roghane gul (oil of Rosa damascene), Safeda (white lead), Sirka (vinegar) and Kafoor *(Cinnamomum camphora)* for ninety days. The study reflected that Unani formulation has significant effect in reduction of Six area, six sign atopic dermatitis (SASSAD) severity score ($p<0.01$) and there was definite reduction in the cardinal symptoms of eczema (Siddiqui *et al.*, 2010).

Clinical efficacy of Unani formulation on eczema

The formulation contains Henna *(Lawsonia inermis)* and Black Cumin *(Nigella sativa)* studied on thirty patient of eczema. After the treatment, improvement in macules, papules and vesicles was 75% with improvement in scaling, lichinification, hyper pigmentation and excoriation. The efficacy of test drug on subjective parameter of eczema was found clinically and statistically significant (Nawab *et al.*, 2008)

4.9 Jarb (Scabies)

Jarb is a skin disease characterised by intense itching particularly during night. Its aetiology is attributed mainly to the fasade dam (blood impairment) produced by a damvi madda (sanguineous matter) intermixed with a safravi madda (bilious matter) or balghame shor (acidic phlegm) (Tabri, 1997). The actual pathogenesis lies in the production of hiddate dam (abnormal heat in blood) due to which blood becomes more viscous and gets shifted towards the skin leading to the formation of papules/vesicles accompanied with itching and exudation (Qamri, 2008). It is mostly found in those people who take excess of salty and sour food items and poor people including labours who bath after prolonged intervals (Maseehi, 2008).

Efficacy of polyherbal Unani formulation

An oral administration of formulation containing *Fumaria indica, Swertia chirayita, Tephrosia purpurea, Sphaeranthus indicus* and *Ziziphus jujuba* along with local application of Sulphur, *Letharg* and *Cinnamomum camphora* was investigated on 30 patients of scabies. After 15 days of treatment, it was observed that out of 30 patients, itching was relieved in 50% cases, pruritic lesions were completely healed in 40 % of cases, skin scrap test was completely negative in 83% cases and burning sensation was relieved in 43% cases (Ali *et al.*, 2006).

Unani drugs tend to be more promising in the field of dermatology as already described by reputed Unani physicians. They have vividly discussed skin diseases, clinical manifestations and treatment in their treatises. The dermatological disorders examined were acne, scabies, eczema, psoriasis, ring worm, urticaria, vitiligo, pityriasis and melasma. In most of the studies Unani medicine was found to be quite effective viz. Acne, (Quamri *et al.*, 2009, Lone *et al.*, 2011, Tabasum *et al.*, 2014, Ara *et al.*, 2014, Sultana *et al.*, 2015), although there were limited studies on pityrasis and scabies (Ali *et al.*, 2006, Lone *et al.*, 2012). None of the studies found that Unani drugs either worsened the condition or had negative effects. Of all outcomes evaluated, the strongest evidence exists to support the efficacy of Unani medicine for improving symptoms of acne. Although the results of our review are encouraging, with most studies displaying a positive effect, the review has several limitations. Though our search strategy involved both electronic and non-electronic data, we may not have identified all the available trials involving Unani drugs. As noted above, most trials were of short duration (4 to 6 weeks), with relatively small sample sizes (n = 30 – 40).These factors prevent us from drawing firm conclusions about the effects of Unani medicine on health outcomes related to skin diseases. Other limitations of the studies in this review include a lack of long-term follow-up, use of single self-report outcome measures, reliance on self-report measures, and lack of moderator analysis. The small sample size most likely precluded the examination of important moderator variables (*e.g.*, gender, age).

In all of the trials included in this review (n =20), among a total of participants, there were no significant adverse events, adding to the safety of Unani medicine. In summary, Unani medicine has vast traditional uses. It has demonstrated efficacy in treating skin diseases; however, a limited number of high-quality clinical trials exist currently. Larger scale randomized controlled clinical trials are needed for better understanding of Unani medicine's potential. Data regarding safety, effectiveness, and mechanisms of action from longer-term trials are needed so that Unani medicine can be widely recommended for the better management of skin diseases and associated disorders. The commonest used drugs among them were blood purifiers. Blood purifiers are broadly defined as group of drugs that remove toxins and waste matter from the blood by diverse mechanism and have been used in Unani system of Medicine since ancient times for treating numerous diseases including blood, skin, spleen and liver disorders. The medicinal properties of blood purifiers are attributed to its physico chemical properties (hot dry temperament, bitter taste) (Qureshi, 1998) and chemical constituents viz. alkaloids, flavonoids, saponins, tannins etc. present in the drugs, which have been found to have strong hepatoprotective, antioxidant, anti allergic, anti microbial, anti septic, anti anaphylactic activity, immunomodulatory, anti fungal, hypoglycemic and anti inflammatory activities (Chauhan *et al.*, 2013).

Products Available in Market for Skin Diseases

Eczema/ Fungal Infection:

Marham Quba, Marham Hina, Roghan Gundum, Qurse Asfar, Eczimo.

Acne:

Gaza Husn Afza, Roop Nikhar, Herbal Face Pack, Herbal Kalonji Oil, Zamad Muhasa.

Boil/Urticaria:

Arq Murakkab Musaffie Khun, Sharbat Musaffie Khun, Habbe Musaffie Khun, Arq Ushba, Arq Mundi, Safi, Khun Safa, Arq Sheer Murakkab, Arq Murakkab, Mauljubn, Ushban, Marham Hina, Musaffie Ajeeb, Neem Cap, Rakt Safa, Marham Kafoori, Musaffie Azam, Khoonseer Majun, Musaffie Khas, Sharbat Khana Saaz, Arq Chob Chini.

Scabies:

Qurs Asfar, Safi, Jerbin, Dawa E Kharish Jaded, Roghan Kameela, Marham Kharish Jaded, Khoon Safa, Safuf Kharish, Arq Sheer Murakkab, Arq Mauljubn, Arq Musaffie Khun, Ushban, Marham Hina, Majun Musaffie Azam, Musaffie Ajeeb, Mausaffie Azam, Rakt Safa, Marham Kafoori, Jarb Khas, Khoonseer, Zamad Jerb, Shabat Khana Saaz, Majun Musaffi Khoon, Arq Chob Chini, Jugnu White Ointmwnt.

Leucoderma:

Safuf Bars, Barsina, Barsina Roghan Babchi, No Bars Ointment, No Bars Tab, Herbal Kalonji Oil.

Wound:

Sanjeevan Tel, Marham Kafoor, Ezay, Heal Cap, Marham Raal, Marham Kafoori, Oleo Hayat.

Burns:

Sanjeevan Tel, Oleo Hayat.

Syphilis:

Jauhar Muanqqa, Majun Musaffie Khas, Habbe Lemu, Majun Musaffie Azam, Marham Atishk Jauhari, Cap Jauhri, Majun Ushba, Kushta Gaudanti, Habbe Suzak, Suzaki, Arq Rahat Khas.

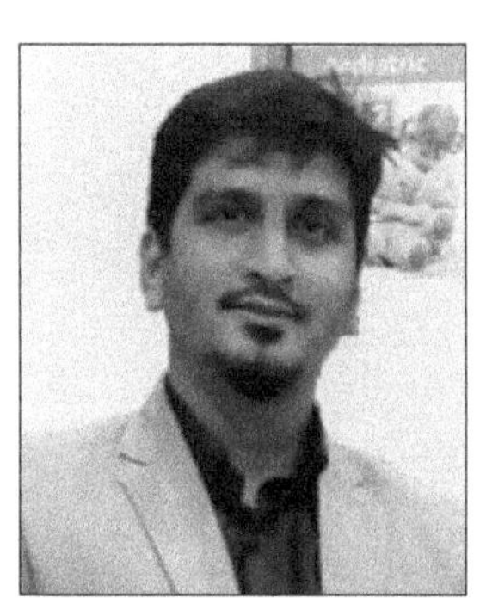

Dr Ansari Mushir

9967660883

ameenhealthcare@gmail.com

www.ingramcontent.com/pod-product-compliance
Ingram Content Group UK Ltd.
Pitfield, Milton Keynes, MK11 3LW, UK
UKHW062311290726
14090UKWH00018B/1006